PENGUIN BOOKS

PACKING IT IN THE EASY WAY

A successful accountant, Allen Carr had a hundred-cigarettes-a-day addiction that was driving him to despair until, in 1983, after countless attempts to quit, he finally discovered what the world had been waiting for – the *Easy Way to Stop Smoking*. He has now built a network of clinics that span the globe and has an unrivalled reputation for success in helping smokers to quit.

Get details of your nearest Allen Carr clinic by calling 0800 389 2115 or visit www.allencarreasyway.com

D0542225

Packing it in the Easy Way

ALLEN CARR

PENGUIN BOOKS

OTHER PENGUIN TITLES BY ALLEN CARR

Allen Carr's Easy Way to Stop Smoking (1987)
The Only Way to Stop Smoking Permanently (1995)
Allen Carr's Easyweigh to Lose Weight (1997)
How to Stop Your Child Smoking (1999)
The Easy Way to Enjoy Flying (2000)
The Little Book of Quitting (2000)
Allen Carr's Easy Way for Women to Stop Smoking (2003)

To Joyce and Serendipity

Also, special thanks to Tessa Rose for her patience and perseverance in the unenviable task of making what I have written readable.

PENGUIN BOOKS

Published by the Penguin Group
Penguin Books Ltd, 80 Strand, London WC2R 0RL, England
Penguin Group (USA) Inc., 375 Hudson Street, New York, New York 10014, USA
Penguin Group (Canada), 10 Alcorn Avenue, Toronto, Ontario, Canada M4V 3B2
(a division of Pearson Penguin Canada Inc.)
Penguin Ireland, 25 St Stephen's Green, Dublin 2, Ireland
(a division of Penguin Books Ltd)
Penguin Group (Australia), 250 Camberwell Road,
Camberwell, Victoria 3124, Australia (a division of Pearson Australia Group Pty Ltd)
Penguin Books India Pvt Ltd, 11 Community Centre, Panchsheel Park, New Delhi – 110 017, India
Penguin Group (NZ), cnr Airborne and Rosedale Roads, Albany,
Auckland 1310, New Zealand (a division of Pearson New Zealand Ltd)
Penguin Books (South Africa) (Pty) Ltd, 24 Sturdee Avenue, Rosebank 2196, South Africa

Penguin Books Ltd, Registered Offices: 80 Strand, London WC2R 0RL, England

www.penguin.com

First published by Michael Joseph 2004
Published in Penguin Books 2005

010

Copyright © Penguin Books and Allen Carr, 2004
All rights reserved

The moral right of the author has been asserted

Typeset by Adam Renvoize
Printed and bound in Great Britain by Clays Ltd, Elcograf S.p.A.

ISBN-13: 978–0–141–01517–0

www.greenpenguin.co.uk

MIX
Paper from
responsible sources
FSC
www.fsc.org   FSC™ C018179

Penguin Books is committed to a sustainable
future for our business, our readers and our planet.
This book is made from Forest Stewardship
Council™ certified paper.

Contents

Preface

Twenty years ago I was a man in crisis. I had all the trappings of success and yet felt undermined and insecure. For over thirty years I had lived with an addiction I loathed and knew was slowly killing me, from the inside out. It is an addiction shared by millions of people, perfectly legal and benefits nobody apart from the big multinationals that manufacture it and the governments that milk it for taxes. My addiction held me in almost total thrall, and no matter how hard I wriggled to get off its hook, time and again I failed, each failure increasing my feelings of personal worthlessness. I tried every method of quitting and called on every inch and ounce of willpower I possessed, all to no avail.

What finally got me off that hook was not my own ingenuity, but an entirely fortuitous happening: my discovery of a method of quitting smoking that I would call Easyway. I knew that my discovery had important implications. It was not a cure personal only to me; it was a cure for all smokers. I wanted to take it out into the world and introduce it to the thousands of smokers who were still stuck in the same pit I had escaped from. Many of the people I have been privileged to help quit smoking have been generous in their estimation of me. But how can anyone be given credit for an accidental discovery, in my case for being touched by serendipity one hot July morning?

Recently I read somewhere that the technique we know as dry-cleaning was discovered because a man accidentally knocked over his paraffin lamp. When some of the liquid spilled onto a grubby tablecloth, he noticed that the impregnated area was visibly cleaner than the remainder. Was he the first person to spill paraffin on a tablecloth? Unlikely. Thousands, possibly millions had done so before him. But he was the first to turn that genuine accident into a valuable discovery. I did the same with Easyway, and for that I am proud to take the credit.

This is the story of how it happened.

Part One

The Hard Way

Earliest Memories

My earliest memory is as a two-year-old lying on my father's chest while he slept in an armchair. I can recapture the rise and fall of his chest and the smell of stale beer on his breath as if it were yesterday. Why I've never forgotten that incident remained a mystery to me until very recently, when I began to look back on my life. A significance attaches to that earliest of memories, although there is no way either of us could have been aware of it at the time. That was the closest I ever got to my father either physically or emotionally.

I have read many books about famous people whose lives seemed to be spent trying to avoid the shadows cast by dominating parents. Perhaps I was lucky in that my parents weren't famous and nor did they offer themselves as examples to be emulated or outshone. My problem has always been trying to live up to my own expectations.

We lived in a lower working-class area of Putney, a suburb of south-west London, whose sole claim to fame is that the annual Oxbridge boat race starts from Putney Bridge. Dad was a self-employed builder and decorator. His hobbies were drinking at the local, betting on horses and chain-smoking. The only time he came on holiday with the rest of the family, he brought his mates with him. As they all shared his hobbies to the exclusion of other more family-friendly leisure pursuits, you can imagine what sort of holiday that turned out to be.

Dad was not an ambitious man. Self-employment was not chosen as a way forward but was the only way forward when he couldn't find anyone prepared to take him on as an employee. His business was lucrative, and yet he was content to use a barrow to trundle his work gear through the streets of Putney. He never did buy a van. I knew him for over a third of a century, and lived in the same house for 20 of those years, but I never really knew him. In fact I can count on the fingers of two hands the specific memories I have of him, and most of those are not particularly pleasant.

However, most kids love their father. I know I respected and feared mine. As a ten-year-old I used to love working with him. I remember the first time I was allowed to climb the ladder to paint some gutters. After five minutes I caught my sleeve in the hook holding the paint tin. It hit the ladder on the way down, spilling its contents everywhere. He and I spent the rest of the day removing green paint from the yard, fence and next door's patio.

He didn't say a word. Nor did he when I managed to block Putney High Street for half-an-hour with a barrow-load of bricks. It had been my first day out pushing the barrow. I had a wide-brimmed trilby hat on, just like his. I felt 6 feet tall until a gust of wind took my hat off, I let go of one of the barrow handles to retrieve it and the load tumbled off. On both occasions his anger would have been preferable to the ensuing stony silence.

The only time he laid a hand on me was at the annual dinner ritual one Christmas. As usual he arrived back late from the pub, drunk, and as usual my mother started to nag him. On this occasion he lost his cool and threatened to strike her. I was already a schoolboy boxing champion and stepped in to protect her. I thought I'd have no problem handling a drunk but he sprung at me with surprising speed and agility. I was helpless. He had his hands round my throat and there was murder in his eyes. I can only speculate that there must have been a look of horror in mine because immediately he released his grip and his temper subsided.

Another of those early memories was of my older sister and her friends wanting to take me to the cinema on a Saturday morning. Ungrateful little brute that I was, the more they tried to cajole me, the more I dug my heels in. Eventually they gave up and went off without me. I was convinced they were bluffing and that they would soon be back trying to persuade me again. Once it dawned on me that they weren't bluffing, I decided I wanted to go. This incident provided my first insight into my character, and probably my mother's too. Throughout my childhood she seemed always to be one step ahead of me.

The quintessence of my mother's attitude to life is summed up by a rhyme which, framed and hand-written in beautiful script, occupied the prime position above our living room fireplace.

'When burdened with worry and life goes wrong, just buckle your armour and trudge along.'

She viewed life on this earth as nothing more than a period of penance to be endured. Worse, she did not believe that her penance would be rewarded in a better life hereafter.

Considering her upbringing, it would have been a miracle if her attitude had been different. The eldest of fourteen children, she had an alcoholic mother and a father who deserted them. While still a child, she had taken on the responsibility of being both mother and father to those children during the worst years of the Depression. There is no doubt whatsoever that my mother's attitude had a profound effect on me and my siblings; my older sister Marion and two younger brothers, Derek and, the baby of the family, John.

Our father appeared to be not so much a person as a zombie. When he wasn't out, he used to sit in front of the fire, reading his newspaper, never conversing. Possibly because we children had ginger hair, he seemed to have difficulty telling us apart. When the inevitable rumpus occurred, my mother would say to him: 'Will you speak to these boys?' I give credit where it is due. He knew our names. He also knew the chronological sequence in which we'd been born. But he didn't know which ginger-haired little brat was the cause of each particular rumpus. He would merely shout: 'Allen! Derek! John!' By admonishing us all, he had chastised the guilty party, discharged his duty and could now return to his newspaper with a clear conscience. It was probably because of his attitude that it didn't seem to matter to us whether we were Allen, Derek or John.

These contributions and the occasional grunt were the extent of my father's participation in family life. This left our mother as the dominating force. I can't remember her holding proper conversations with us either. Try to imagine a regimental sergeant major communicating with a subordinate. Even when addressed to an officer, his words will be delivered in a loud, clipped and decisive tone that in no way could be described as conversational. Like all ranks faced with such a monolith, we children were never either courageous or stupid enough to hazard ideas that might contradict hers.

Such were our parents. Our father made no attempt to talk to us and she didn't know how. I loved her dearly, and I knew instinctively that she loved me, although I was the bane of her life. Frequently she would threaten to put her head in the gas oven because I was so naughty. Although I didn't realize it at the time, I was – and possibly still can be – contrary. There's a Benny Hill sketch that sums me up in this respect.

Teddy Boy: 'I don't like being accused.'

Interviewer: 'That's understandable, but were you guilty?'

Teddy Boy: 'Yes, but I don't like being accused.'

I was in a similar predicament. Whenever there was a rumpus at home with my brothers, my mother would rush in and proceed to whack me. Invariably I was the cause of the rumpus, but my mother would never bother to enquire what it was all about before she meted out punishment. I could cope with the whacking. It was the injustice of no trial or inquisition that I found unbearable.

The indifference of my father on the one side and the threats and whackings of my mother on the other would nowadays probably have child psychiatrists hastily scribbling case notes on the dire consequences of leaving me in such a household. If my upbringing has had adverse effects on me, I've yet to feel them. Violence defined as a smack is said to breed violence. I cannot agree. There are about five incidents in my life that I would change if I could do so. One of those five incidents was that I once slapped my youngest son. He doesn't remember the incident. I can never forget it.

I thought our situation at home was normal. In those days in the area where we lived, it was. It was normal for the man of the house to spend every night in the pub and for the mother to struggle to feed and clothe the children. It wasn't until I went to grammar school and came into contact with children from a different background that I began to question what is normal.

Initially I regarded the parents of these other children as really weird. The fathers would actually spend their evenings at home, and they appeared to be genuinely interested in how their offspring were getting on at school. The mothers didn't appear to be aggressive and permanently under stress. Fathers and mothers would talk to their children as if they were human and didn't view them as infant monsters they had been cursed with.

The subject of my parents is still a live topic of conversation for my brothers and me, as it was with Marion until her untimely death at the age of 56. Perhaps because there is a space of only three years between each of the four of us, our impressions of what life was like then and how our parents were are remarkably similar. None of us feels that we really knew them. It was quite a shock to learn, much later, that my father had been the life and soul of the party at the pub when surrounded by his friends. My younger self had blamed him for his absences, but perhaps he had chosen that course as preferable to permanently removing himself from our lives. Later I would come to appreciate how difficult it is to live with somebody who is almost constantly depressed. My mother could not be blamed for being the victim of her upbringing, but nor could my father for taking refuge elsewhere in order to cope with its consequences.

Whatever their faults, they gave me the most precious gift that any of us can possibly receive – life. Be they the most humble and unimpressive parents that ever gave birth, for that alone I thank them. Whether intentional or otherwise, the whackings, indifference and the like, prepared me for a wonderful and productive life. Certainly, they ensured that I have never taken anything for granted. I have received with gratitude life's gifts and tried to make the best of its burdens, which thankfully have been remarkably few.

The Outbreak of War

The outbreak of the Second World War was by far the most significant event of my early years. It was 3 September 1939, the day after my fifth birthday. Although I was far too young to understand what it was all about, it was impossible not to be contaminated by the atmosphere of overt excitement tempered by unspoken fears. Derek, Marion, our pregnant mother and I were immediately evacuated to Reading. My father stayed behind, newly elevated in our eyes as a full-time fireman. I remember being given a banana sandwich just before boarding the train and being told that there would be no more bananas until the war was over. It turned out to be true. There was even a ridiculous song: 'Yes, we have no bananas'. Even to this day my favourite food is a banana sandwich.

My mother convinced me that the war had only started because I was naughty. I felt very guilty for all the trouble I had caused. I still believed her tale years later, even when it must have been obvious that she hadn't been telling the truth.

I'm grateful that I had little understanding of the true gravity of the situation. I had been indoctrinated to believe that England, and London in particular, stood at the centre of the universe, that the British Empire was invincible, that Britain ruled the waves and that we Britons never, never would be slaves. The first blow to my belief in British supremacy had come when I learned that Joe Louis, the world heavyweight boxing champion and my hero, was not British but American. It came as an even greater shock when a week later I found out that he was not only an American but a black American. The only black man I had ever seen was the local road sweeper. All other impressions came from Hollywood films, and they were hardly flattering. There was no Harry Belafonte, Diana Ross, Sidney Poitier, Dorothy Dandridge or Mohammed Ali. But, for a small, ignorant boy infatuated by sport, Joe Louis alone was enough to help explode the myth of the superiority of the white man.

After the initial excitement wore off, evacuation was not much fun. Marion and I were billeted about a mile from my mother and Derek, with a couple who were as poor as they were unfriendly. I got the strong impression that we were wanted only for the money that giving us a roof over our heads attracted. Later mother arranged for us all to be billeted together in a large detached house where we had the top floor to ourselves. The house was next door to a bakery, run by a Yorkshire couple. They were the kindest most easygoing people I had yet to meet. I was allowed to assist in the baking and Marion, Derek and me would spend hours playing with the couple's three sons. In nearby Salmon Wood we would pick bluebells and primroses and collect chestnuts and firewood. This was my first taste of the country, and I loved it. To the local ruffians, however, we were known as bomb-dodgers. Sticks and stones may break my bones but names can never hurt me. But at that vulnerable age names are far more painful than a bloody nose. I believed myself to be a bomb-dodger and a coward and did not question the stupidity of the accusation.

Reading introduced me to the noble art of self-preservation. School was about a two-mile walk from our billet. There was a choice of two routes. If I took the first I could be sure of three comparatively minor skirmishes. The second was a short-cut inhabited by a particularly vicious individual who was two years older and a foot taller than me. In the first few months I opted exclusively for the first route and became nimble and adept at slipping punches. I became quite pleased with myself, and for the first time questioned a belief instilled in me by my parents that you were either born with a natural aptitude for a particular activity or you weren't. The smile on my face was soon wiped off my face when I reached school, where my consistently late arrival was attracting the unwelcome attentions of my teacher. The pen is said to be mightier than the sword. That teacher taught me that the tongue can be mightier than the other two put together.

One particular morning I started out late and, fearing an even worse verbal battering than usual, decided to risk the short cut. The monster was laying in wait, salivating at the mouth because I had starved him for so long. From a distance I had regarded him as the natural successor to the legendary Brown Bomber. Up close I discovered the limits of his potential. He didn't land one punch on me, although it wasn't for want of trying. I was so quick and elusive that he was made to look like a clod-hopper. From that day on I always took the short route and the monster gave me a wide berth.

This was probably the earliest example of serendipity in my life. Had I not been late, I would not have been introduced to a very important lesson: that bullies are large, empty bubbles. Prick them and they will explode.

After spending about a year in Reading we returned to London briefly, before being dispatched again, this time to Kettering. I was billeted on my own, with a couple who had a son about three years older than me. Although they seemed quite prosperous, my abiding memory of living in their home is of feeling ill at ease. I used to suffer from nosebleeds. One in particular was very bad and occurred while I was staying with them. The bleeding began at four in the afternoon and was showing no sign of stopping at eight in the evening. By this time I was also vomiting, caused by swallowing the blood. When my mother arrived with a doctor, the landlady assailed them with complaints about the mess. This incident decided my parents that we should move back to London permanently. The worst of the Blitz was over, and risking the danger of flying bombs was preferable to living apart in the homes of people who did not want us.

We children spent the rest of the war collecting shrapnel from bombed-out streets. The doodle-bug suddenly cutting out overhead or the bomb whistling past were exciting events, never mind that either might fall on us. The flattened houses belonged to other people.

We were regular attendees of Sunday school, not for our religious enlightenment so much as to allow our father to sleep off the effects of the booze and the weekly roast in peace. The only difference between school and the Sunday variety was the day of the week. I can't remember how old I was or the occasion when I stopped believing in Father Christmas but I would have been quite young. Exploding the myth of God was another matter. I never believed there was an omnipotent being judging my every action, but the indoctrination to do just that was powerful. With all the adults around me insisting on perpetuating the myth of God while readily dismissing the existence of Father Christmas, the upshot was doubt and confusion in my mind. How could they believe in one myth but not the other? The only constructive response was to make mischief, which I did so successfully that I was asked to leave Sunday School and not return.

I was a typical street urchin, as were all my friends. I was aware that I wasn't educated and mistakenly believed education and intelligence to be one and the same. At each of the different schools I attended the teachers merely confirmed what my mother had already taught me – that I was a naughty, cantankerous child. I learned to master the basic principles of reading, writing and arithmetic, but that was about it. At 10 years of age a dark shadow began to loom over our lives in the shape of the 11-Plus. The teachers made us aware of its importance. Certain that I wouldn't pass, I didn't let their premonitions bother me.

Then something remarkable happened: I passed. What's more, on the strength of it I was invited to attend the local grammar school in Wandsworth, Sutherland Grove. I imagined myself as some latter-day Tom Brown. Although they never admitted it, I'm sure my parents were as shocked as I was.

The Best Days of My Life?

The exhilaration of being invited to attend a grammar school quickly evaporated when on bragging to my fellow street urchins I discovered that half of them would be going too. It turned out that we were part of the new social experiment following the war whereby every child got an equal chance in education, irrespective of social background. However, much of the old prejudice remained, and was reinforced by the streaming system operated by grammar schools. At one extreme was the A form, consisting almost entirely of boys who hailed from the more refined areas in the immediate locality. At the other was the C form, consisting entirely of street urchins. In the middle was the B form, which included me and was a combination of urchins with a little more savvy than the rest and the upper crust who were too thick to be in the A form.

The knowledge that I was not a genius had its compensations. One of the fears of changing schools is that you will be separated from your chums, and it was comforting to find several of them with me at Wandsworth Grammar. In no time at all, however, I was mixing in different circles, although I was never consciously aware of dropping any of my old friends, or of deliberately trying to cultivate new ones.

When we first arrived at the school we received an extended introduction detailing what a wonderful place it was and how lucky we were to be there. But no one explained exactly why we were there. Yes, we understood the general objective was to accumulate knowledge, although learning Shakespeare and algebra did not strike us as particularly helpful to our future lives. I've yet to meet a single person who found a use for algebra in later life. The excuse proffered was that it developed intelligence. It struck me as extremely unintelligent not to give us the opportunity to study subjects that would be of practical use as well as develop our intelligence. I learned Boyle's law and Ohm's law parrot fashion without having a clue as to their meaning, yet left the school five years later incapable of changing a fuse or wiring a three-pin plug. Understandably we formed the general impression that we were there for the same reason we were sent to Sunday school – to keep us out of mischief until we were old enough to work.

It was the teachers' function to infiltrate our brains with knowledge and it was the function of the kids in my stream to ensure that none of it got through. We were more united than the most solid of trade unions in this respect. All our efforts went into playing truant or games like battleships and cruisers. Even then we couldn't outdo C stream. A stream were another matter, a bunch of weirdoes, softies and bookworms who not only didn't resist the indoctrination but seemed to revel in it. Given these differing attitudes, it was not surprising that you remained in the stream you started in. You might go up a form or stay put, depending on your results in the annual exam designed to test the amount of knowledge each of us had accumulated, but bucking the streaming system was another matter. As luck would have it, I did manage to migrate from B to A through no extra effort. An inordinate number of boys from the A and C streams left the school during the fourth year, either due to expulsions or a desire for private cramming before the GCE exams, and so the numbers in the three streams had become unbalanced. On the suggestion of my housemaster it was agreed that I should be moved to the A stream.

On reflection, I have no doubt this event was by far the most important and influential in my life. In the B stream I was a king, and proud of the reputation I was building as a tearaway. I'd already been to juvenile court for stealing ball bearings from an army depot, and was heading for a life as a dropout and petty criminal. I hated going into the A stream and protested bitterly at my exile. In one fell swoop I had lost all my friends and found myself surrounded by a bunch of aliens.

Up until this point, the one redeeming feature of the school had been the emphasis on sport. Although short and light for my age, I was already a boxing champion. It wasn't that I enjoyed the sport – I hated it – but I liked what I was told went with being good at it. The male of all species, we were told, was basically an aggressive animal with an innate desire to fight. The noble art of self-defence was a way of channelling that aggression, building character and sorting out who got the pick of the girls. My instinctive desire to be admired by the female of the species was the strongest factor motivating me to excel. Certainly I did not have the slightest inclination to fight other males for the sake of it. I had no desire to inflict punishment on them and was positively horrified by the prospect of them doing likewise to me. Another motivating factor was fierce inter-house rivalry.

I gather that at every public school one house seems to take the lion's share of the prizes and accolades. At Tom Brown's Rugby it was School House, which must have made the boys of the other houses wonder whether they belonged in the same institution. At Wandsworth Grammar the chosen house was Cromwell. The others were Gibbon, Pitt and, my house, Morley.

The cream of the annual intake was put in Cromwell, which produced all the Old Wandsworthians who went on to make names for themselves. Cromwell always had more boys than any other house, and because a point was awarded just for entering a competition, it always won more than its fair share of the points. Naturally, when there were intra-school competitions the boys from the other houses wanted any house but Cromwell to win.

One of the five events in my life that I cannot reflect upon without despising myself occurred in the final of an inter-house boxing competition. I was up against a close friend, a boy called Jimmy Coppack, a Cromwellian. Jimmy was no boxer and in the days leading up to the final he had several times emphasized what good friends we were. I pretended that any friendship would be on hold from the moment the first round bell sounded. Secretly I intended to hit him with enough light blows to earn an easy points victory. By the end of the second round the match had become more like an exhibition of shadow boxing than a serious fight.

I arrived back in my corner with a holier-than-thou feeling, only to be greeted by a tirade from my second: 'What's the matter with you? While you're pissing around, Jimmy's winning on points!'

This was serious. The point-count between Morley and Cromwell was finely balanced. It hadn't occurred to me that while I was pulling punches, I wasn't landing them. Jimmy wasn't pulling his, and he was. When Jimmy came out for the third round, the fear had gone from his eyes. He believed I had no intention of pulverizing him. Up until this point I hadn't, but the thought of Cromwell actually winning the cup and beating my house swept all consideration of his preservation from my mind.

Jimmy was tall for his weight and a bit gawky. He came out for the final round, jaw agape. I hit it as hard as I could. I can still see his spittle projecting across the ring. Impregnated even more indelibly in my mind is the look in his eyes, and the thought behind it: 'You bastard! You had no need to do that!'

Morley won the cup. Had Cromwell triumphed, I've no doubt that I would have suffered recriminations for a few days, even weeks. As it was, I am still reproaching myself 55 years later.

Apart from boxing, I was also good at cricket and rugby. I captained the school junior rugby and cricket teams and was selected to play for Surrey against Kent juniors in both sports. Some of the other boys in A stream were also interested in sports, notably Jimmy Nelson, who was to be a great influence on me. Jimmy's background was very similar to mine and he lived within a mile of my home. There the similarities ended. Our attitude to life could not have been more different.

At some of the important crossroads in our lives, our options are extremely limited while at others we have a choice of several. Jimmy was unlike any of my former street-urchin friends who, to a boy, had always looked after No. 1. If Jimmy had an orange, he would share it. Such generosity was completely unknown to me. Jimmy also gave me my first experience of the superiority of intelligence over physical aggression. Confronted by a thug who was not prepared to accept an apology for being accidentally bumped into, Jimmy stood his ground, not the least fazed by the other boy's attitude or impressive bulk. While he smiled up at him and calmly enquired, 'What's your problem?', I was calculating whether we should hit him first and then run, or just run. Neither was necessary. The other boy backed down, and we continued on our way.

This example stood in stark contrast to what my mother had demonstrated to my eight-year-old self, after I had complained of being bullied by a local boy. She had dragged me outside by the collar and made me hit him back. Jimmy's approach made the deeper impression.

I have described how the sole objective of the pupils in the B and C streams was to ensure that knowledge didn't permeate their brains. When I arrived in the A stream, I discovered that some teaching methods could transcend even a deliberate attempt to remain ignorant. Known – among other things – as 'Ascher the Basher' and 'Ascher the Thrasher', Mr Ascher helped me to get a distinction in French, and in the process taught me how to cope with verbal bullies. In appearance he was like a jovial version of Topol, except that he was about five feet tall and approximately the same in circumference. To each new class he would explain that in the thirty years he had spent preparing students for GCE, he had never achieved a single pass. It turned out that he had never had a single failure either – just credits and distinctions. In my particular year, a class of 22, there were 5 credits and 17 distinctions.

His French lessons were a nightmare. One pupil would be asked to read a question from his book to which the pupil behind him had to answer in French. At the slightest mispronunciation or error he would puff up like a bullfrog about to explode, frothing at the mouth and his face turning purple. Then he would not so much walk as vibrate towards his victim. We waited in vain for him to have a heart attack, and confronted by his unfailingly robust health turned to devising other measures to escape his wrath. One plan was to calculate in advance what our question or answer would be. This worked so long as no one botched an answer and Ascher asked him to read the next question. To safeguard against this, we took to writing our anticipated answer down on a piece of paper, which would be passed to the person sitting in front so that he was covered. However, an expert persecutor is always one step ahead of his victim, and Mr Ascher must have come across every permutation of cheating that schoolboy minds can devise. The moment we started passing the answers, he would reverse the sequence.

Ascher terrified me. I coped by the simple expedients of keeping my head down and becoming good at French. One boy, Totham, had the measure of him and would remain unperturbed even when facing his worst mouth-foaming moods. The rest of us did not dare to adopt Totham's technique of sitting there, grinning at him. Clearly Ascher thought there was a danger of his authority being undermined and Totham was eventually moved to the B stream. Totham showed me how to handle a windbag, but I would wait until I was the same size as such antagonists before following his example.

My schooldays were characterized more by boredom than happiness. I wasn't unhappy so much as disengaged from the whole process. This attitude prevailed until my final year when, motivated by the thought of getting a well-paid job, I studied and crammed furiously in order to pass a string of GCEs: maths, French, geography, history, English grammar and English literature.

Just before sitting those exams we received lectures from accountants, solicitors, stockbrokers and the like. I still can't believe my naivety. I thought these people were genuinely interested in our future and had come to give us impartial advice. The reality was they were there to attract the cream to their own business or profession. On their part the teachers were there to ensure we upheld the function of the grammar school system, which was to get us into respectable professions. We were being equipped to become lawyers, bankers, doctors and accountants, certainly not plumbers, electricians or bricklayers. At no stage was it even hinted at that we might do better working for ourselves or following career paths unrelated to the professions.

I can recall a talk given to us by a banker. Actually, that's not strictly true. What I remember is him telling us how much we would earn as bank managers, and being very impressed by the figure. In those days £1000 per annum was a very handsome salary. Banking, the man told us, equipped the individual like no other profession and gave insights into other careers. He would be pleased to answer any questions we had. One boy took him at his word and asked what would be the chances of him becoming a groundsman. His question was entirely serious. He loved sport and he wanted to do something in that line. The response was suppressed laughter from the teachers and rowdy guffaws of derision from the other boys. The bank manager was flabbergasted. Clearly, the message regarding the purpose of a grammar school education was not getting through to all-comers.

The guardians of our future, the teachers, were not interested in us on an individual basis either, and probably had a hard job telling us apart. Mr Aubrey was a classic example of the worst sort: pompous and eager to humiliate. Fortunately, my contact with him was limited, but on both occasions he left a mark. The first was on the rugby pitch, where he was determined to demonstrate the validity of his claim to have been a Welsh international. I suppose it was optimistic to expect my under-five stones frame to bring down all fifteen stones of his in one tackle. After launching myself at his bulk, I struggled to encircle one of his thighs with my arms. I clung on to that thigh for a few seconds in the firm belief that he would fall over in admiration at my bravery and tenacity. Instead, he swatted me as if I were a fly, brushed aside the other five-stoners in his path and dived over the line as if he was scoring a winning try at Cardiff Arms Park.

I settled the score a bit later. The occasion was a heavy snowfall. The school building was fronted by two playing fields and as each master entered the gate he had to run the gauntlet of boys waiting to ambush him with snowballs. All accepted the loss of their dignity in the right spirit and legged it to safety as quickly as they were able. That is, all but Mr. Aubrey. He stood in the entrance, pulled himself up to his full height and bellowed:

'The first boy to throw a snowball at me won't even live to regret it!'

In those days, masters were not only allowed to beat children, they were expected to, and would have been considered as failing in their duty if they did not. They were part of a vicious circle of discipline. If your parents found out you'd had a caning at school, you were more than likely to get another when you got home.

To 11- and 12-year-olds Mr Aubrey cut a very impressive figure, head held erect, jaw jutting, confidently staring straight ahead, but at the same time looking ridiculously pompous. Still smarting from the tackle incident, I let rip. My snowball hit him squarely on his left eye. He didn't flinch. But the spell was broken. Snowballs rained down on him from all directions. He remained motionless for about 10 seconds before putting his head down and taking to his heels. I was expecting severe retribution. It never came, probably because he did not know who I was. As it turned out, Mr Aubrey would more than get his own back without being aware of it.

The day of reckoning was pencilled in three or so years later, when I was sent to him for careers advice. This made little sense, because he had never taught me and knew absolutely nothing about me personally. At the end of our very brief session together, he said,

'Carr, you are good at maths. I strongly recommend that you become an accountant.'

I had no idea what being an accountant entailed, and at this distance I'm convinced Mr Aubrey hadn't either. Our combined ignorance would result in my entering a profession that I would end up hating.

The four credits and two distinctions I got in the GCE examinations were enough to get me into accountancy. University had not been an option, even if I had wanted to go. My parents informed me that my housemaster – Mr Benyon – thought I wasn't brainy enough. The truth came out many years later, when my mother told me that I had matriculated but they could not have afforded to send me. She thought she had acted for the best.

Jimmy Nelson and I were of a mind that university was merely an excuse for boys who were afraid to leave school and go out into the real world. And we couldn't wait to go.

I'm Going to be a Chartered Accountant

My parents were clearly impressed by the future marked out for me, although they had no clearer picture of accountancy than I did, other than that figures were involved. My dad thought it might be very useful when taking the chalk during a game of darts.

I was regarded as very fortunate to receive articles from Peat, Marwick, Mitchell & Company, one of the 'big five' accountancy firms with branches throughout the world. Aged 15, I started off as an office boy, making tea, running errands and generally dog's-bodying. The large, dusty, old-fashioned office was straight out of Dickens and I pictured myself as Bob Cratchit. I loathed it. After six months I was given what was presented as a promotion, except that it wasn't accompanied by an increase in salary. I was put in the general services department where, apart from delivering letters and parcels, my most responsible job was to stick stamps on envelopes, and this I learned to do at least ten times faster than the standard rate.

Although I resented the work, which bore no resemblance to a training in accountancy, the experience was worthwhile. The office was run incredibly efficiently, and I had to apply myself to whatever menial tasks were handed down. The head of the department, Mr Marshall, a chronic alcoholic, had nothing whatsoever to do with this efficiency, which was due entirely to his assistant Skinner, an incredible man whose type I have only ever encountered in films. On celluloid he would have been the tough sergeant-major who is a mother and inspiration to the lower ranks, wise counsel to the young officers and right-hand man to the colonel. Skinner managed to keep me out of Marshall's way and ran that office rather as a circus performer spins plates on a hundred bamboo sticks. I never saw Skinner drop a single plate and I never heard him get a single word of praise from Marshall or anyone else whose life he made easier.

After another six months it dawned on me that the firm would be happy for me to carry on licking stamps and boots until kingdom come. By now I'd begun to glean the sort of work I should be doing in order to become a qualified accountant. I had to threaten to leave before the firm agreed to transfer me to an auditing department.

Audits were carried out at the premises of the companies whose accounts we were engaged to check. Most of these offices were located in London's West End, which was a far more exciting location for a teenager than the City. Occasionally we had to travel to locations in other parts of the country. Our clients, ever mindful that we might discover some huge error in their books, would treat us like lords and, where necessary, put us up in the best hotels.

Many of my fellow articled clerks were lords, or at least sons of lords, and in the main ex-public schoolboys who had been trained to expect to be the leaders of men. Although the same age as me, they were mature, confident young gentlemen who were used to dining in the finest restaurants, knew the correct wine for each course and thought nothing of sending the bottle back if the contents did not come up to expectations. Jo Lyons' self-service was my idea of the ultimate in gourmandise. I compared myself with those young men and felt like a pimply oaf.

My first experience of auditing out of town did nothing to boost my self-confidence. One of our biggest clients was the British Electricity Authority, or BEA as everybody referred to it. I was told to get a train to Portsmouth and take a taxi to the company's offices, which were quite near the station. After half an hour in the taxi the meter reading exceeded the amount of cash I had on me. On querying the driver he pointed out that I had asked for BEA and he was taking me to British European Airways at Southampton. I thought it was the sort of thing that could happen to anybody, but my boss had no difficulty in convincing me that it could only happen to an oik like me.

When eventually I turned up at the right BEA, the only irregularity I uncovered was operated by the man in charge of the audit. There was an arrangement with the hotelier, he told me, whereby we received two bills, the lower of which we paid and the higher on which we claimed our expenses. I refused to go along with this deception, determined that my brush with the law over the ball bearings would be my one and only. I was told I had to comply, otherwise head office might notice the disparity between my bill and the bills submitted by my colleagues. I had no intention of informing on them but I refused to be implicated. In the end we found a compromise. I stayed in a more expensive hotel.

It was inevitable that sooner or later my decision not to become a smoker would be challenged. I hadn't smoked since my first experience of cigarettes at the age of ten, when I had gone thirds on a packet of five Woodbine with two other street urchins. Then I had struggled not to throw up, while insisting through the fumes that my cigarette tasted very nice. Had the remaining two cigarettes been oranges we would have been fighting over them, but with untypical generosity each of us had insisted that the others should have them.

This incident should have kept me free for life, but like most people I under-estimated the power of nicotine. I was auditing at a firm in Biggleswade with a chain-smoker called Ron Gazy when I got hooked. Every time he lit up, he would offer me a cigarette and I would have to remind him that I didn't smoke. Now Ron had a very sharp brain. No way could anyone accuse him of being absent-minded and yet somehow he never seemed to remember that I didn't smoke. I don't believe he deliberately tried to get me hooked, and to this day I have no idea whether he was just being polite or whether he was ameliorating the uncomfortable feeling that lone addicts tend to experience in the company of non-addicts. Eventually I capitulated. The audit wasn't going very well and it seemed like an act of solidarity to smoke too. I sensed that Ron needed a fellow smoker. In his turn Ron seemed to appreciate my gesture by continuing to proffer the ever-open packet. Gradually cigarettes became less obnoxious and I was able to accept more frequently. Although you could say that I had learnt to cope with cigarettes, in no way was I under the impression that I enjoyed them or was in danger of getting hooked. One morning, as I accepted the first of the day, Ron joked:

'You keep smoking my cigarettes! When are you going to buy a packet?

I was indignant. 'Buy! What idiot would pay good money for these filthy things? I kept telling you I didn't smoke, so why did you keep pushing them on me? I was doing you a favour!'

That's what I wanted to say, but of course I didn't. For years I believed that the reason I kept my mouth shut was to avoid upsetting him.

Ron's comment stung me into making that first purchase, and from then on I was careful to keep my offers in step with his. The notion that my actions were shaped by a wish to help someone else out in the first instance and then to avoid hurting their feelings in the second was the kind of self-deception that most smokers indulge in. I could have offered Ron the occasional cigarette without smoking myself. After this experience I vowed to myself that I would never accept other people's cigarettes or buy them for myself.

By the time of my next out-of-town audit, I was well and truly in the nicotine trap, smoking heavily and believing that I needed cigarettes to help me concentrate.

The Latest Craze

The only aspect of school I missed after leaving it was the sport. I wasn't alone, and so with a few friends I would play cricket or football, according to the season, on Putney Common. These forays did much to compensate my ego for the battering it received at work.

However, one by one these friends began to drop out until only two of us were left – Jimmy Nelson and me. Neither sport is much fun with just two players, and so we looked around for alternatives. Jimmy was all right – he was an accomplished pianist and a great jazz fan. I had no such talent or interest and, reluctant as I was, felt I had no choice but to follow the example of my friends and join them in the latest craze – girls.

I'd enjoyed the usual games of doctors and nurses as a child and at the age of ten I had fallen in love for the first time with a girl in my class, Jean Warner. But girls didn't seem interested in playing football or cricket and, sport fanatic that I was, I counted that as a drawback to friendship with them.

In those days our hobbies were dominated by the cinema and changed every week. When *Robin Hood* was showing we were blinding each other with bows and arrows. With *The Thief of Baghdad*, kitted out with towels on our heads and blankets round our shoulders, we spent our days jumping off walls. *Tarzan* sent us swinging through trees on ropes in our swimming costumes. But my downfall was brought about by Mark Twain's Tom Sawyer or, more precisely, his girlfriend Becky. I loved those characters. Becky had red hair, and it was because of Becky that I fell in love with Jean. She had the most gorgeous head of red hair reaching half-way down her back. So blinded was I by her personification of Becky that I overlooked her bland personality, and the fact that she was teacher's pet, neither of them characteristics I admired.

But the hair had it, and I was smitten. My courting technique in those days was somewhat limited and consisted of laying in wait for her with a bunch of friends and then pushing one of them into her as she passed. After five years at a boys' school, obsessed with sport and, later, passing exams, my approach failed to attract the interest of sophisticated 15-year-olds.

My reluctance to be part of the girl craze was in part due to current trends in cinema heroes, and my own sense of myself. Before adolescence I had swashbuckled, swung from branches and beaten my chest with the best of them. It had all been fun. Now on the verge of manhood I felt awkward, sensing that more was expected of me. I couldn't attempt to ape the leading men of the day. Clark Gable, Tyrone Power, Cary Grant, Gregory Peck and Walter Pidgeon were all TDH – Tall, Dark and Handsome. I was less than average height, ginger and decidedly ugly. Several people told me I looked like singer Matt Monroe. I'm sure they intended the comparison as a compliment, but as much as I loved his voice, I disliked his features.

So there I was: short, ginger and ugly, whose only tried courting technique was to push his friend into the path of the girl he fancied. This was before the days of discos. However, we had one great advantage over today's youngsters. It was called ballroom dancing. This was before the liberated Sixties, when a girl was regarded as somewhat risqué if she let you kiss her on the third date. Yet amazingly, it was quite acceptable to hold her in a clinch on the dance floor and place your groin firmly against hers. Not only was this position acceptable, but you weren't regarded as a good dancer unless you adopted it.

The trouble was, I couldn't dance. I got my sister to teach me the basics of the waltz, but my first outing came before I'd learned to reverse or to avoid other dancers. As you can imagine, it was a disaster, as were my next few forays. One of the worst aspects was the system, with the boys on one side of the room eyeing the girls on the other. Without doubt my bravest act has been to cross that great divide and ask a girl to dance, in the sure knowledge that if she refused no way would another girl accept my invitation.

I became a keen observer and noticed there were several boys shorter and uglier than myself who not only had many partners but were popular in the dance I most dreaded : the ladies' invitation. I also noticed that several TDHs were wallflowers. I worked out that provided you were not shorter than the girl, she didn't care how short, ginger, ugly or lacking in conversational skills you were. If you were a good dancer, no girl would refuse you. Physical attraction didn't come into the equation. What the girls wanted was your skill as a dancer to show them off and make them more attractive to the boys they were interested in. None of them would take the floor with a carthorse that would drag them down to its level. I set about becoming a good dancer.

I calculated that what I needed most was practice. But the business of asking girls to dance was such an ordeal that I'd remain firmly stuck in the carthorse stage unless I could find a way round the problem. Emboldened by the occasion of a dance at my old school, I invited a local girl who seemed to have trouble getting boyfriends. I wasn't a particularly good dancer, I explained, with stunning understatement. To my amazement, she accepted. My plan was brilliant: I'd calculated that if I paid her entrance fee – the princely sum of two shillings and sixpence – she would be honour-bound to dance with me most of the evening.

However, just as the best laid plans of mice and men can go astray, so did mine. True, we did have the first dance. If I'm honest, it probably wasn't the most exciting dance she'd ever had. As her luck would have it, a particularly good-looking TDH took a fancy to her and she spent the rest of the evening dancing with him. I couldn't blame her. He was not only a TDH – in looks he was Britain's answer to Jimmy Stewart – but a good dancer as well. I wrote the half-a-crown off to experience.

They say it's an ill wind that doesn't blow somebody some good. This particular ill-wind turned out to be nothing less than a treasure chest that has endowed me with pleasure throughout my life. The morning after the dance, that particular TDH rang my doorbell and apologized profusely for pinching my girlfriend. It turned out that he was also an old Wandsworthian and had been in the same year as me but in the C stream. Over fifty years later and now a TGreyH, Desmond Jones is still a firm friend.

Our relationship was a microcosm of life. I'd started at the grammar school with a king-sized inferiority complex and finished as a sporting hero. At school Desmond had been a skinny non-entity. Now I was a pimply, gormless carthorse and he was my hero: a sophisticated TDH, who danced like Fred Astaire and had a chat-up style that would have made Erroll Flynn envious. Apart from chasing girls, the main thing we had in common was a very keen and somewhat distorted sense of humour. In the girl department, he was the master and I was his devoted pupil and learned very quickly. He introduced me to dancing lessons at evening classes and to a local Church-sponsored social club where I met my second embodiment of good fortune.

Her name was Doreen Wright, but everyone knew her as Dodo. Only fifteen and still at school, she was the nearest that we could get to a top American cheerleader. Already she had a figure like Marilyn Monroe's and the most fascinating flashing green eyes. She loved to be surrounded and admired by men. I got a look in because she was mad about dancing. The TDHs were slightly too tall for her and couldn't show her off to best advantage. I was already becoming a competent dancer, and physically she and I were the perfect meld. I was very fit and more than happy to bathe in her limelight as she tore around the dance floor completing all sorts of gyrations and variations. She introduced me to the delights of the Hammersmith Palais, where each Sunday morning the best ballroom and Latin-American dance instructors in the world would give lessons. Unbelievably, both entrance and lessons were free. Once I became Dodo's regular dancing partner, ladies' invitations became a bind rather than a nightmare.

I have Des and Dodo to thank for helping me to realize that my adolescent pimples were imaginary and that I wasn't condemned to be a carthorse forever. Socially, my life was perking up considerably, but at work I was still the ignoramus trying to hold his own against the natural leaders of the land.

Calling the Tune

For most boys of my generation National Service loomed up like some giant cloud to blank out our fun. I saw it as an escape from the nightmare I was living as an articled clerk. But first I had to pass the strict medical examination. I was a sports fanatic, incredibly fit, and the thought that I might not pass it never entered my head, even though my friend Desmond had already been declared unfit due to contracting TB. At the time TB was regarded very much as cancer is today, with dread. Part of the medical involved a chest X-ray. It came as a great shock to receive a letter which informed me that my X-ray was unsatisfactory and that I needed to see a specialist.

I feared that I too must have succumbed to TB. Although my mother said nothing, I could sense she was even more worried than I was. I duly turned up to see the specialist only to be told there was a fault in the X-ray rather than in my lungs and that I was fit to join the RAF. I breathed a huge sigh of relief and went home to share the news with my mother, before going into the backyard to play a game of one-a-side cricket with brother Derek. After only a few minutes I had completely dismissed the episode from my mind. I wasn't going to die of TB, end of story. The most important challenge facing me as my father walked through the back gate was beating Derek.

My father made no apology for interrupting our game, but he did have the good manners to ask how it went. I was most surprised, because he'd never taken any interest in our matches before. I started to explain that I was over a hundred ahead on the first innings. He said: 'I'm talking about your X-ray!'

It's only now, as I reflect upon my life, that I understand the significance of that moment. Then I didn't have the wit to read it properly, otherwise I could have built on his gesture and made the effort to engage with him. Up to his death and beyond I regarded him as completely indifferent to what went on in my life or how I felt. I misjudged him, as did all of his children.

The prospect of spending two years away from Peat Marwick was an exciting one. Ken Young, a fellow articled clerk at Peat Marwick, had just completed his National Service and was full of insights about what I could expect. His first tip was that I should try to collect as many female pen-friends as possible. This I did, and by the time of my official posting, I had accumulated promises from a dozen attractive girls to write to me regularly. According to Ken, provided you survived the initiation, life in the RAF could be like living in a holiday camp, a veritable paradise on earth.

The reception camp at RAF Padgate turned out to be a dismal place and left me with a distorted impression of the climate in the north of England which would linger for years. Reveille was at 5am, whereupon the doors and windows of the Nissen huts housing us were thrown wide open, letting in the ever-present mist. We were then marched through the murky blackness to the cook-house. Although a haven of light and warmth, it promised far more than it ever delivered. The term cook-house seemed a misnomer and did not adequately describe what was actually done to the food. Bacon, to name but one victim, was so burnt that it would explode into a thousand inedible fragments on being pierced with a fork. Like every other recruit, my surplus cash – the little I had managed to save before going into the services – was spent on chocolate bars in the NAAFI. My mother helped to alleviate the dietary shortfall by sending regular food parcels. Every Friday we would line up to receive a meagre weekly wage of 28 shillings. By Tuesday most recruits were broke and were begging or borrowing funds on which to enjoy the weekend.

I was already smoking roll-ups before I went into the forces because I couldn't afford ready-mades. Knowing that I faced a further reduction in income, I had intended to quit smoking the moment I joined up, but those initial weeks were so unsettling, I decided to put off the evil day. It wasn't long before the need for tobacco had extinguished the few extra pounds I had taken with me. There was no question about it, I would have to start selling off my assets: a smart Ronson lighter, cigarette case, Rolls razor and my watch.

After Padgate I was sent to a square-bashing camp at Hednesford near Wolverhampton, where I learnt how to load, fire, clean and strip a rifle and how to march in step. The drill was by far the most important part of our training and entailed not only doing the manoeuvres correctly but looking good. At Hednesford I discovered that the 1952 intake did not consist entirely of 18-year-old conscripts such as myself. It was liberally sprinkled with WW2 veterans who had failed to adapt to civilian life, and hard nuts who had joined up from front lines as diverse as Glasgow's Gorbels and London's East End.

I was prepared for those eight weeks being a living hell. Our drill instructors – or DIs as these corporals were commonly known – ensured I wasn't disappointed. They pranced about the square like prima donnas, made virtues of bad-temper and unreasonableness, and held to a particular sartorial style with almost religious fervour. The creases in their trousers could have been used to carve a joint of beef, and the shine on their boots was blinding. The slightest speck of dirt or dust on our clothing or equipment would send them into paroxysms of fury. Incapable of speaking in a normal tone of voice, they would deliver their venomous tirades in demonic, high-pitched screams. The ogre with the vicious tongue was still alive and very well.

I was terrified, as I had been earlier when confronted by the formidable and unforgiving teachers of my school years. I had not the slightest desire to rebel. I wasn't alone. The WW2 vets, several of whom had won medals for valour, and the hard nuts instinctively knew better than to get on the wrong side of these banshees. National Service did not teach discipline, as many have claimed, as much as recognition of the paramountcy of self-preservation. Each hard nut, war vet and 18-year-old concentrated on becoming the archetypal invisible man.

When our eight-week stint of square-bashing was nearing its end, we had to decide how we were going to occupy ourselves for the remainder of our stay in the forces. It was like the end of my time at Wandsworth Grammar all over again, only now we were being persuaded to become grease monkeys, pay clerks, or electronic wizards. None of these occupations appealed to me. At an advisory session one of the officers suggested that we might want to become drill instructors.

It seemed like some sort of sick joke and, there being no DIs present, we hooted with laughter.

But he wasn't joking. He explained that the training consisted of eight weeks at RAF Uxbridge, and that only a quarter of the applicants could expect to complete the course. I hardly heard the last part and couldn't care less about completing the course. The magic word Uxbridge sold the idea to me. It was at the end of the Piccadilly Line, just an hour from home, my friends, Dodo and all those other lovely girls, and handouts. I would no longer need to eke out meagre supplies of tobacco by making up increasingly frail roll-ups.

Apart from the rather dubious ambition of becoming a chartered accountant after the completion of my National Service, I had no immediate aims other than to tackle each week as it came and survive the course for DIs. Twice I was in danger of being thrown off it. Both times I had to plead with the Squadron Leader in charge to allow me to remain. My first misdemeanour had been to go to a dance in my boots and not give myself enough time to 'spit and polish' them to the required standard before parade the following morning. My second was to allow my hair to grow beyond the regulation short back and sides. I had tried to delay paying for a proper haircut by the simple expedient of shaving the quick-growing hair on the back of my neck. The parade sergeant claimed my hair was so long that he was standing on it. I played up to his exaggeration, explaining that a rash on my neck caused by a blunt razor had prevented me from getting my hair cut. I never expected the Squadron Leader to accept this explanation, but he did.

You don't see adverts offering six-figure salaries to ex-RAF drill instructors. The best you can hope for after such training is a job as a night watchman or security guard. From my perspective, the experience it gave me was invaluable, most importantly in terms of the insights it allowed into the make-up of a type of person that up to this point in my life had always got the better of me: the wind-bag.

When I became a DI I was automatically cast in the role of demi-god. Unlike the worst demi-gods, I was not self-anointed. The system did the anointing for me. I just wore the uniform and behaved as DIs were expected to behave: loudly and seemingly as automata. I mastered the banshee wail on the drill ground, the impeccable attention to detail, and the sarcastic humour.

Now I find it difficult to believe the reverence shown me in my guise as a DI, even as an 18-year-old trainee when, before passing out from Uxbridge, I was involved in drilling officers for the Coronation celebrations. I took no great delight in bellowing, and certainly did not aspire to be as scary as the men who had put me through my paces as a rookie. No way could I have actually become like them. I was too aware of who I really was beneath the play-acting. I was not alone. The other DIs were just like me, average guys playing a part to the best of their ability.

My experience as a DI taught me that people will accept you for whatever you purport to be. Invariably they won't scratch the surface to find the quivering wreck beneath. In my case I had sufficient self-belief not to quiver and I never knowingly treated my subordinates badly. 'Sticks and stones may break my bones but names can never hurt me' is one of the earliest maxims we chant as children. It would pay us to really believe it. I'll wager the majority of us spend our entire lives unappreciative of this truth, and that many people who like to think of themselves as being physically and mentally strong in most circumstances can too easily be reduced to trembling shadows of themselves by verbal bullying.

Being a DI gave me a hike in rank – to corporal – and wages, and also unexpected scope for supplementing my income. Most recruits spent about two hours each evening polishing their boots to the exacting standard set by us DIs. They all moaned about this chore, as indeed had I until I developed a technique that enabled me to produce sparkling heels and toe caps after only ten minutes of spitting and polishing. I charged 10 pence a pair. There was one essential for any racket to be successful: that it was worthwhile for both parties. As I was the man who inspected the recruits' boots every morning, they were assured of good service. And by giving a good service I ensured that even if the racket was suspected by the commissioned officers, I would never be dropped directly in it by a disgruntled 'customer'.

Trousers were another important item for scrutiny at the morning parade. They had to be neatly pressed and have a sharp crease to pass inspection. When first issued to recruits the trousers were very woolly and therefore very difficult to press. With only one iron per billet and this shared between 22 recruits, there was much consternation and sometimes fighting as airmen struggled to meet the standards expected of them. I developed a technique of shaving off the excess wool and stitching the fabric so that it gave the appearance of having a crease. The recruits in my care were more than happy to pay five pounds to have a permanent razor-sharp crease embedded in their trousers

All the NCOs worked rackets. Mine kept me busy, often into the small hours. Some rackets were better than others in terms of the income generated and the genuine usefulness of the service rendered. I took pride in the fact that mine were doing a good turn all round. The best racket I discovered was another example of serendipity.

New recruits weren't allowed any leave until they had completed their basic training. However on Saturdays and Sundays, when there were no lectures or drill, they were allowed off the base for a few hours if they passed inspection by the duty NCO, who would then hand over their ID cards to enable them to get through the front gate. This was no mean feat. Jobs involving power and boredom tend to bring out the worst in certain types of people, and some of the duty NCOs would amuse themselves by being incredibly pernickety. This would result in a long queue, with each failure sending the recruit to the tail end and in many cases ensuring he wouldn't pass the inspection until it was too late for him to go anywhere. I abhorred this practice as being both unnecessarily cruel and bad for morale. In my experience even the bolshiest recruit was easier to handle if was allowed to spend time relaxing away from the camp.

One particular Saturday a recruit came to me close to tears. He had received a 'Dear John' letter from his fiancée and wanted to get to London to persuade her against dumping him. He had failed the inspection four times and it was now past midday. He was a nice lad and I felt for him. I went down to where the ID cards were kept, took out his card and told him that he had to be sure to get back by midnight on Sunday. If anything went wrong, he did not get his ID card from me. There followed bad news and good. He wasn't able to change his fiancée's mind. However, he did tell other recruits about my role in his escape home. The following Friday I was approached by a Brummie lad who offered to pay me ten shillings if I could get his ID card. Like any good business my reputation spread by word of mouth from one satisfied customer to another.

Prior to my enlistment, my main activity had been to collect as many female pen-friends as possible. The one I had met immediately preceding National Service, I was particularly attracted to. The fact that now I can't even remember her name, let alone what she looked like or where she lived, leads me to believe that the only reason I was so attracted was because I was deprived of her company. Certainly I found no diversions on the weekends I spent out of the camp. The local girls couldn't compete with the beauties I used to ogle routinely each day on the tube journey from Putney to the City. Having to queue up with 20 other airmen for just one dance with the local farmer's daughter increased my homesickness for the Hammersmith Palais and the buzz of the metropolis.

After completing my two years of National Service, I had a choice of whether to join the RAF properly and sign up for several years or make my way back to civvy street. I was sorely tempted to stay and prolong my enjoyment of being a DI. In many respects it was like a fantasy life, in which I was a somebody and treated with remarkable deference by the 22 recruits under my command. I excelled in my role. Every week my platoon would win the prize for best billet and be the leading platoon on passing out parade. It was very seductive and a large part of me railed against the certain knowledge that if I took the other route, I would be welcomed back to my job in the city as a nobody. I felt like an ego-driven Superman contemplating his transmogrification into Clark Kent. But I knew my life as a DI was too good to last. I had to face up to the real world. Deep in my subconscious I probably heard the voice of my mother, urging me to accept responsibility for my future.

I arrived home in Putney a very different proposition from the immature, shy youth that had left two years earlier. It took some time for my parents to adjust to the change and acknowlege that I was now a confident young man.

Those Penny Policies

In the Fifties it was more or less standard practice for working-class families to take out an insurance policy on their lives. Such a policy could be taken out for as little as one penny a week. The man – usually from the Prudential – would call weekly to collect the premium, which averaged about ten pence from each family. In social status he ranked slightly below the local GP, a rating he patently did not merit in terms of the good he did. In reality he was a door-to-door salesman who played on the fears and conscience of poorly paid people who would have been better advised to put their money elsewhere. But in those days not being able to afford a respectable 'send off' was seen as the ultimate indignity.

I'd hardly settled into home life again when my mother informed me that the man from the Pru would be calling round with his supervisor on Thursday evening to see me about taking out a policy. I didn't want life assurance, and resented the assumption that I should blindly follow the example of my parents and their neighbours. My mother could not understand my attitude. Partly to avoid her embarrassment, I agreed to meet them.

They left without my business. My mother regarded me differently after that episode, as did she the man from the Pru, but while I went up in her estimation he went irredeemably down.

I put off the evil day of returning to Peat Marwick until I could put it off no longer. My welcome back into the company's fold was all that I expected. After arriving promptly at 9 o'clock, feeling down and dismal, I spent the next two hours waiting for an interview with a departmental manager. I knew I would be placed in the large general office alongside the other articled clerks and the chartered accountants. The only individuals to merit offices were the managers and under-managers of the various auditing departments.

I spent those two hours observing the people with whom I would be working and becoming re-acquainted with office politics. Two of the qualified men were obviously vying to become top dog. One of them, named Westwood, I had accompanied on an audit. I remembered him as an exceedingly intelligent and pleasant man. It took me some time to recognize him, mainly because he'd lost his pleasant Cumbrian brogue and now sported a bowler, pin-stripes and the compulsory umbrella which, I would discover, was never un-rolled even in the heaviest downpour.

The second man, who I hadn't come across before, named Ingram, had obviously been born with a silver spoon in his mouth. There had already been several minor skirmishes between the pair. Now came the clincher, involving what was, in those pre-Biro days, an accountant's most precious possession – his Parker 51 fountain pen.

Westwood: 'Does anybody have some ink?'
Ingram: 'There's a bottle under your nose.'

Westwood: 'I know! But is it Quink?' *(One up to Westwood)*

Ingram: 'Doesn't it say Quink on the bottle'? *(One all)*

Westwood: 'I know it says Quink, but these bottles are topped up with all sorts of ink.'

Ingram, after walking the full length of the office, picking up the bottle and taking two deep sniffs, proclaimed:

'It's Quink all right.'

I was fully expecting him to hazard a guess as to the year but he was content with his victory and didn't push his luck. No one was amused, least of all me. I had been in the building less than an hour and was already wondering how long I would be able to stand the pettiness and futility of it all.

Needless to say, I persevered. My mother's example and my own experience in the RAF had equipped me for the long haul. In retrospect, I couldn't have chosen a better profession to prepare me for the life that lay ahead. There were three reasons for this. The first involved my co-workers.

There were two distinct types of qualified chartered accountants: former articled clerks who had qualified with the firm, and accountants who had qualified with smaller provincial firms and had joined Peats to enhance their curriculum vitae. Just as parents find it difficult to accept that their offspring are no longer children, so the management at Peats found it difficult to accept that their once gormless office boys and then slightly less gormless articled clerks had blossomed into fully qualified chartered accountants. The men who qualified in the provinces, even those newly qualified, were treated with much more respect than the 'natives'. The 'natives' had experience of auditing the largest companies in the land, whereas the out-of-towners had probably not had much more to deal with than the local farmers' accounts.

That said, the newly qualified accountants who joined Peats for experience were the firm's go-getters. The average audit lasted about two weeks and during that period one of these ambitious young men was my boss. On the next audit, it would be another. I had ample opportunity to compare their techniques and pick their brains.

One of the great pluses of working for a firm like Peat Marwick was that from a comparatively young age I was allowed to share the financial secrets of some of the largest and most profitable businesses in the country. Many of these companies were incredibly inefficient and made money in spite of their organizational shortcomings. They provided important insights into how to run a business profitably and efficiently.

It didn't take long for me to learn that practically every set of accounts presented for audit either understated the true profits in order to avoid tax or overstated them to fool the shareholders and/or bankers. I developed a nose for deception. Typical giveaways were the form of wording chosen, omissions and sometimes even the fact that a company had found it necessary to make a statement about a particular aspect of their business. The ability to read between the lines proved invaluable when later I came to establish the true facts about smoking.

Even though I was finding the work more interesting, I still had no real ambition to become a chartered accountant. I was just going through the motions in the absence of an ambition. I had no particular loyalty to Peat Marwick. Quite the reverse. My negative attitude was not helped by the response I got when I asked for my first pay rise.

That departmental manager who had kept me waiting two hours on my return to the firm was a sarcastic, cynical wet fish of a man called Dunkerley, and it was to him that I had to make my request. It took me six weeks of careful planning before I dared approach him. Just as a chess champion has to anticipate the tactics his opponent might adopt, so I had worked out a counter for every conceivable objection Dunkerley could raise.

On the morning I decided to tackle Dunkerley I noticed a cartoon in my newspaper showing the fate of a man similarly minded.

'No need to tell me,' the dejected man is chided by his wife on returning home, 'I can see that you didn't ask for that rise.'

'I'm sorry, dear. In the excitement of getting the sack, I forgot.'

Although convinced I would share this fate, I had gone past the point of caring. The entire general office knew what I was about to do, and their interest bolstered my flagging bravado. I couldn't back down now. In my determination to appear self-assured, I knocked twice as loudly as I had intended. After a long pause – no doubt intentional and designed to demoralize – my knock was acknowledged with the single command, 'Come'. The addition of the word 'in' was far too much effort for such a self-important man.

Had the watching crowd not been there, I would have walked out and never returned. But they were there and I had no choice but to open the door and walk in.

Dunkerley did not give me so much as a glance, and remained absorbed in the documents on his desk.

Eventually he deigned to look up: 'Yes?'

'I believe I'm being underpaid.'

At this time I was earning about £3.50 per week. The average annual rise was about 25 pence. These sound ridiculously meagre amounts by today's standards but that increase represented nearly 7 percent of my wage.

'How much do you think you are worth?'

So far so good. I had anticipated this line of argument and immediately came back with '£4.50', hoping to settle eventually at £4.00. Instead, he said:

'You're on £4.50 dated back to the beginning of the month', and went straight back to his documents.

I'd got twice the rise I would have been happy with, but did I feel elated? On the contrary, I felt cheated, and chastised myself for not having asked for more. Was that good management? Not in my book. If Dunkerley didn't think I was worth £4.50, he should have refuted my statement. If he thought I was worth that amount or more, he could have obtained my loyalty by giving me a rise, unasked.

Some time later another important watershed occurred, after which, if the firm had asked me to cut off an arm without explanation, I would willingly have done so.

I had recently passed my intermediate exam and, although not fully qualified, was entrusted to conduct audits at clients' offices without being supervised by a qualified accountant. I'd been observing different management techniques and had come to the conclusion that officers, whether in the military or commerce, fell into two broad categories. There were those who tried to disguise a basic lack of confidence by assuming a pompous air and impressing with an attitude which said: 'Your job is to follow my orders and not question them.'

In the other group were those in positions of responsibility because they knew their job. These managers were delighted to explain exactly why what they were telling you was correct. They also appreciated being questioned and took it as a healthy sign of interest.

The company secretary of the first firm I was entrusted to audit alone was a classic example of the first category. His name was Fincham. He had never qualified and clearly objected to a young upstart like me demanding to see his company's books and asking all sorts of questions that he regarded as being none of my business. Fincham had made a science out of making an auditor's life as miserable as possible.

For each audit we were handed a programme or listing of the various accounting books. The books were more or less standard for each company. However, this particular company's audit programme included a book that was new to me, referred to as 'the black book'. Fincham had produced the standard books on request but not this book, nor had he mentioned its existence. Auditors are empowered by law to examine all the books and records of a company, and so I asked him to produce the black book.

It turned out that our manager, Mr Dunkerley, audited the black book personally. Nowhere in the audit programme was this stated and Fincham did not enlighten me on this point, choosing instead to greet my request with an outright refusal. Undaunted, I persisted until it became apparent that he was not going to change his mind. Then I came out with the auditor's ace in the hole: unless you produce that book we will not approve the accounts. This didn't move him either. With a triumphant grin on his face, he said that I'd need to take the matter up with the managing director, president and owner of the firm, Sir Walter Wallace.

Many self-made men at that time seemed as if they had come out of a mould, and Sir Walter was no exception: barely over five feet tall, stocky, booming voice, iron-grey hair and with piercing eyes that, you feared, could see deep inside your brain. He had a huge office with a proportionate-sized desk raised on a two-foot dais, in front of which was a single chair which – I'd swear – had the legs reduced by six inches. That was where unfortunates like me sat. The set-up and Sir Walter's manner had the effect of making you feel as if you'd crawled in under the door rather than walked through it. My confidence was at rock-bottom, even though I knew I was on very strong ground.

Sir Walter began the interrogation, in stentorian tones:

'Mr Fincham tells me that you refuse to sign the auditor's report.'

'Unless we are allowed to see all the relevant information, we cannot possibly be expected to sign it.'

'Sir Harry Peat is a personal friend of mine. I think he'd be interested to know that he's not going to sign it.'

With that he picked up his phone and dialled Sir Harry's number. There were over 30 partners in the City branch of Peat Marwicks, and I had not seen one of them, including Sir Harold Peat, the founder partner, who was also president of the Institute of Chartered Accountants. I'd only seen my manager on five occasions and those included my interview and my request for a rise. Even the junior partners were treated like exalted beings. Sir Harry was about as remote from me as Zeus.

While I deliberated on whether to go back into the services or to try my hand at something else, Sir Walter was barking pleasantries at Sir Harry. Then he got to the nub of the matter:

'Look, there's a slight problem, Harry, which I'm sure you can sort out. I've got your Mr, er, Carr, I think it is, and he tells me you won't sign the audit report!'

He let out a guffaw of hearty laughter, echoed by Fincham, who throughout my ordeal hadn't been able to keep a self-satisfied smirk off his face.

Sir Harry's sobre reply was unequivocal and heard distinctly by all three of us:

'If Mr Carr says I won't sign the audit report, then I won't sign the audit report.'

A stony silence followed the loud clunk of the receiver at the other end of the line.

At this time the business ethos was such that it was not uncommon for lowly employees to be sacrificed to satisfy the egos of valuable clients. The customer was always right. Sir Harry's reaction was untypical. By taking my side and reducing Sir Walter and Fincham to their true stature, he inspired my undying devotion.

Although this incident finally established my loyalty to the firm, it could not spark my interest in the work. The way I looked at it, if I had to earn my living doing something I didn't particularly enjoy, there were a lot worse jobs. And auditing did offer excellent opportunities for meeting attractive girls without having to go to dances. This was a definite plus because the social life I had enjoyed before going into the RAF had largely evaporated. I had expected to return home and carry on where I had left off, and got a nasty shock when it turned out that my friends had got on with their lives in my absence. Desmond was managing a dance hall in Brighton, and of the rest of our crowd some had moved and the others were either married or far advanced in that direction. Imperceptibly but firmly we were all being guided along the path to marriage and child rearing.

Ellen

Ellen Healey was the receptionist and telephonist at a small firm in Wapping. She had perfect features, shoulder-length chestnut hair and a pleasant disposition. My normally ready wit had a habit of evaporating when I tried chatting up girls. This didn't happen with Ellen, who possessed the charming ability of being able to talk with ease for long periods without requiring any contribution from the person she happened to be conversing with. Not for a moment did I think she had her eye on me, because our conversations consisted almost entirely of her telling me about her problems with previous or current boyfriends. Despite the absence of an apparent personal interest in me, I eventually plucked up the courage to ask her out. I had taken the plunge on the basis of nothing ventured nothing gained, and didn't expect her to accept, but she did. Nine months later, we married.

If you are surmising that the period of our courtship was significant, you would be wrong. Even in those days a salary of £8 a week could not support a wife and baby. Children were out of the question until I had qualified. In the interim Ellen would be subsidizing me.

Under the terms of my articles I had to obtain permission to marry from the partner to whom I was articled at Peat Marwick. This was Mr Nicholson, an exceptionally pleasant man I regarded as a bit of an old fogey. He must have been all of 45. How our perspective changes as we grow older.

I thought Mr Nicholson's approval would be a mere formality but, nice as he was, he took his responsibilities very seriously and asked me how we would manage if we were 'blessed with a child'. I felt like asking him if he had heard of birth control and telling him that modern couples no longer needed to leave such matters to chance. I explained that we were two intelligent, young but mature adults, and were completely in control of our finances and libidos.

Neither would prove to be strictly the case. Our finances were decidedly shaky, so much so that I had tried to avoid buying Ellen an engagement ring, deeming it an unaffordable luxury. When it had become clear that she had set her heart on having one, I relented. I didn't have any savings and so had to squeeze the cost out of my salary. I stopped smoking and rationed myself to a meat pie and a cup of tea from a stall. When I had accumulated £20, I bought her a ring. To her credit, Ellen had been delighted. The penny had dropped in my brain when she showed it to her younger sister, Maureen. After staring at the trophy hard for several minutes, Maureen had cried scornfully: 'You can't see it!' 'It' was the minuscule diamond fighting for visibility. I had considered £20 quite a sum, but of course it didn't buy much in the way of gems.

Hurt by the suggestion that my sacrifice had not been good enough, I went straight out and bought a packet of cigarettes. Maureen had a cruelly truthful turn of phrase, but at base she had a kind heart, and for two years after our marriage she let us share her flat in Wapping virtually rent free.

Wapping was Ellen's home territory. Lying at the heart of London's docklands, it was an area in decline. All around were the remnants of a once thriving port, derelict wharves and warehouses overrun with weeds and rats. It would be thirty years or more before anyone had the bright idea of reinventing the area as a home to the newsprint industry and well-heeled City types who wanted conveniently situated penthouses with river views.

I had been used to Putney, surrounded by common land and beautiful Richmond Park, and found Wapping a dark and depressing contrast. Because the old docks were enclosed by high walls and there were few exits, there was a pervasive sense of isolation from the neighbouring districts. No buses ran through the area and access was mainly via the tube station. In those days few people could afford cars. The station was situated immediately adjacent to the Thames, and its walls literally dripped with water. Ellen assured me this was purely condensation but I was never able to remove the conviction that the walls were about to cave in.

I'll never forget my first visit. I stepped off the tube train looking like a Persil advert, dressed in a smart suit and presenting a gleaming white shirt front. No sooner had the tube departed than a steam train came hurtling through, instantly transforming me into the sad individual who wasn't using Persil. However, the station did serve to prepare the optimistic visitor for what was to come. Directly outside was the main street, consisting of grimy warehouses, blocks of drab council flats, one pub, one cafe and a newsagent. This was Wapping circa 1956.

To be fair, it had one important feature that made the two years I spent there tolerable. Probably because of its isolation, a genuine community spirit had grown up and enveloped all those who settled within its bleak walls. The Wappingites were tough and not to be crossed, but they were also very friendly and outgoing.

Most of the residents were descended from Irish immigrants, both Catholics (Catlicks) and Protestants (Prodidogs). Each religion organized its annual procession, as opposed to march, through the streets and both events appeared to be cause for celebration by the whole community. Inter-marriage and friendships across the religious divide were quite common. The people themselves had less of a problem with this inter-mingling than did the authorities. Ellen's mother was Church of England and her father Roman Catholic. At least he was until after some years of marriage blessed with six children the local priest asked him when he was going to renounce the woman he'd been living with. He decided to renounce his religion instead.

Shortly after our arrival in Wapping I sat and passed the Intermediate accountancy exams. Ahead of me lay three years of studying for my Finals. Married life combined with Wapping helped to keep me focused. While my friends were out most evenings enjoying themselves, I had my head down studying subjects I loathed. Lack of money helped keep my nose to the grindstone, as did the fact that the nightlife on offer did not extend beyond the depressing.

Many people think that accountancy is concerned principally with number crunching and working out mathematical formulas. This is far from the case. At Peat Marwick anything mathematically complicated was handed over to specialist comptometer operators. The core of the work involved knowledge of myriad aspects of law – statute law, equity law, case law, common law, commercial law, company law, executorship law, intestate law, bankruptcy law, liquidation law and mercantile law. Mastering the basic mathematical principles necessary for qualification gave me a few sleepless nights, but at no time did I doubt their relevance or the logic invested in them.

What attracted me to mathematics as a child was its firm establishment of principles. Once you learn that 6 times 7 equals 42, for example, you need never worry about it changing: 6 times 7 will forever equal 42. You can depend on mathematics – it does exactly what it says on the packet. It came as a grave disappointment to find that the same could not be said of the law.

There's a joke about a man who advertised for the services of a one-armed accountant. Asked why he had specified a one-armed accountant, the man explained, 'Every time I ask my existing accountant a question, he says, "On the one hand you could do such and such, but on the other hand ..."'

After poring over my textbooks for months, I understood how such jokes came to be made.

One case I studied concerned a man who made a will in the expectation of dying of cancer and then died of pneumonia. The question was whether the cause of death being different rendered the will null and void. I thought the answer was obvious: the man would bequeath his property in exactly the same way whether he died of cancer or pneumonia. The precise nature of the illness that carried him off seemed irrelevant. Not so, according to the law. Further reading revealed that this decision was turned over in the High Court and then reversed again at the Court of Appeal. The whole process seemed like building a home on quicksand with the poor layman never sure of when he was on firm ground.

The mathematical side of accountancy was scientific, logical and exact. That I enjoyed. The legal side was unscientific and often appeared vague and illogical. I found it difficult and frustrating to reconcile the two aspects.

Being expected to accept wisdom that seemed deeply flawed made studying doubly difficult. This would not have been so bad if I thought there would be an end to my studying, but this was far from the case. The laws whose details I had to absorb were in a state of constant flux. This was especially true of taxation. Not a year would go by without the Chancellor's tinkering resulting in yet another change. All I wanted was to qualify, learn my trade, and make a reasonable living out of it. I did not relish the prospect of spending the entirety of my professional life striving to maintain a high level of expertise in subjects I loathed. That I persisted even as far as qualifying was, on reflection, due entirely to my mother's influence. I felt burdened but could not bring myself to put that burden down. Somehow I would cope.

Coping financially involved making sacrifices, especially when a few months after moving in with Maureen we discovered that Ellen was pregnant. One of my contributions was to revert to eking out a meagre supply of loose tobacco in anaemic roll-ups. I allowed myself two ounces of Golden Virginia tobacco a week, which made up to about five packets of twenties. Stopping smoking completely was out of the question. I had to have my fix of nicotine. There were also opportunities for doing freelance taxation work for acquaintances. When our finances were particularly shaky, I was prepared to take on anything legal, including agreeing to act as a photographer's assistant at the wedding of an old school friend of Ellen's. I have one vivid memory of that event.

At the reception Ellen's friend told me just to ask at the bar if I needed a drink. When eventually I did, her father, Mr Jones, who was running the bar, greeted my request for a gin and tonic with a look of surprised hostility.

'What yer doing 'ere?' he growled. Immediately the surrounding chatter ceased, my shoulder was grasped from behind in a grip of steel and I was pulled around to face the largest, ugliest brute I'd ever laid eyes on. He stared at me hard for what seemed like an hour but what was probably only a couple of seconds before pronouncing me of no account.

The tension in the air evaporated as quickly as it had gathered and the socializing carried on, as though such interruptions were the norm. I got my gin and tonic but no apology. It turned out that I was initially suspected of being a member of the Kray gang, which was a rival outfit to that run by Mr Jones. The vetting had been done by a South African called Bobby Ramsey, who was on the run from a murder charge in his own country.

In the mid-Fifties the Kray twins, Ronnie and Reggie, were building their empire of extortion in the East End. I had never heard of them before I moved to Wapping, nor of their counterparts like Mr Jones who lived as criminals and yet belonged to the communities in which they operated. People 'in the know' were aware of which pubs were the haunts of the various rival gangs. I went out drinking so rarely that I had not bothered to discover which of them to avoid. One misty evening my friend Desmond came over to take me away from my studies and Wapping. We headed for the neighbouring district of Shadwell. As we drove slowly around in his old Ford, searching for a decent pub, a man stepped out in front of us as if the car didn't exist. Des gave a warning toot of his horn, at which the man stopped in the middle of the road and glared at us before casually completing his crossing. A few minutes later we spotted a pub that looked respectable and pulled over. Inside were two adjoining bars, one of them empty; the other was the venue for a card school. I ordered a couple of drinks and we settled at a table in the empty bar. When we were ready for another round, Des got up to place our order and I sat listening to the animated voices of the card players. I was about to go over to see what they were playing when who should appear but the jaywalker. I stayed put. There was something about him that made me feel apprehensive. He said nothing, just stared for a few seconds before going into the other bar.

Moments later one of the card players came up to where I was sitting and announced in a low, menacing tone, 'We want this table.' It didn't take a Sherlock Holmes to weigh up the situation and conclude that it would be prudent to leave. The messenger was obviously expecting and hoping for some resistance. When I replied pleasantly 'No problem, be my guest', he stood there, brain stuck in neutral, showing all the signs of someone unused to exchanging the usual civilities. I joined Des at the bar to find that our pints had already been poured. He protested when I told him we were leaving. There wasn't time to explain or argue: 'If you haven't drunk up in 30 seconds, I'm going to pick you up and carry you out.'

The tone in my voice must have persuaded him of the gravity of the situation. Following my example, he downed his pint in a time that students in training for a drinking competition would have been proud to equal. Some years later I recognized the jaywalker from a photograph in a newspaper. His name was Ronnie Kray. Needless to say, we did not make a return visit to that pub. A short time later we moved out of the area altogether and made a new home for ourselves in Putney, with our son, John. The biggest hurdle facing us now was my final accountancy exam.

I felt relaxed about it beforehand, but everything that could have gone wrong during it did. At one stage I was about to throw in the towel and walk out. What prevented me was recollecting something Ken Young, the man who had prepared me for the delights of National Service, had told me. Finding himself in a similar predicament, he had resisted the impulse to give up and had taken himself in hand: 'If I can just hang in there,' he told himself, 'I might not have to endure this ordeal a year later.' I too struggled on, although convinced that my perseverance would not bring its own reward.

Confirmation of my fate would not be received until six months later. I knew the exact date I could expect the result. On that May morning Ellen and I sat waiting for the postman. We lived at the bottom of a hill and each day the postman would appear at the top and work his way down to us. In those days you could set your watch by the time the postman shoved your mail through the letterbox. Ken Young had told me that you didn't even need to open the envelope to know the result. If it was thick, you could rejoice. If it was thin, chances were that you would have to go through the ordeal again.

Normally the postman would only stop at three or four houses before he reached ours, but on the vital day he stopped at every one. Finally he approached our house, extracting a single letter from his post-bag as he did so. I asked Ellen if she thought the envelope was thick or thin. Usually a very decisive person, she could only offer that she thought it was 'sort of medium'. I was of exactly the same opinion.

A few seconds later, it dropped onto the mat. We stared at it for some moments before I summoned the courage to pick it up. A few more moments elapsed before I opened it. The discovery that I had actually passed that exam had us both dancing around the room, on my part out of sheer relief. What I experienced was 'sort of' exhilaration. Failure would have been so much worse but it was impossible to experience pure joy over something that of itself meant so little. Passing that exam and being qualified simply meant we were financially secure. I hoped it would mean we could now enjoy our lives to the full.

Most newly qualified accountants aim to start building an impressive curriculum vitae. It was usual to spend about four years gaining post-qualification experience in the profession before either setting up a practice of your own or buying a partnership in another firm. I remained at Peat Marwick. There I was involved mainly in auditing, and preparing accounts and tax returns, all tasks I loathed. Those days would have been unbearable without the refuge provided by another dimension to my life, beyond work and indeed beyond my young and growing family.

Des and I had first gone to Richmond public golf course to do battle with the little white ball when I was studying for my intermediate exams. He had walked away from the game in disgust after just one round, whereas I had been captivated. From that day on it took root at the centre of my social life. Weekends I spent almost entirely on the golf course. Much of the pleasure of the game was that it took me outdoors and gave me much needed exercise. The years I had spent studying and being bound to a desk had eroded the incredible fitness I had built up during the period of my National Service. Bodily I had become prematurely middle aged, a process that was not helped by my chainsmoking. As well as enabling me to look my age, golf, particularly while I was at Peat Marwick, made my life more bearable. I would sit at my desk, pen in hand, seemingly engrossed in a ledger, whereas in fact my mind would be a world away from the tedium and pettiness of my working day, analysing my previous round or planning the next.

By the time I qualified the clear leader in the field of general office politics was a man named Brian Aungiers. He had gone so far in staking out his superiority over the rest of us as to clear out a small junk room next to the assistant manager's office and make it his own. In time he also arranged to have the desk of the department's secretary-cum-typist moved to immediately outside his office door. Newcomers got the distinct impression that she was primarily Aungiers' secretary but that other people were allowed to use her services whenever he didn't require them.

Aungiers was a very shrewd man, and an expert in the game of bluff. It was impossible to prove him wrong, even when you knew he was. I burnt the midnight oil on more than one occasion to find evidence that would support an argument against him, but he was never to be bested. Infuriating though he was to work with, he did inadvertently teach me a lot about office politics, which would stand me in good stead later.

A valuable corrective to the influence of Aungiers was provided by Mr Benson, Peat Marwicks youngest ever partner outside the family. On completing an audit for which you were responsible it was standard practice to be interrogated by your manager and then by a partner. My only contact with Benson came after one such audit. I was fully expecting him to be a souped-up version of Aungiers, and framed my answers to him accordingly. I was particularly pleased with the way one answer was going because of its convolution and inclusion of several long and impressive-sounding words. Mr Benson cut me off in mid-sentence:

'I'm sorry, but I haven't understood a word you've said. Would you mind starting again and please treat me as the biggest idiot you've ever met, using words of one syllable wherever possible.'

I was flabbergasted – and deeply unimpressed – that someone with Mr Benson's reputedly brilliant mind should need to be treated like a simpleton. Eventually, after spending much time pondering the matter, I recognized the value in his approach. Sure the bluff and bravado of Aungiers are useful in certain situations, but they are a great handicap when you are trying to learn or understand something. How many pupils are frightened to put their hands up in class and say, 'Please sir, I don't understand' because they dread the sarcastic remark and the mockery of their classmates? Most people go through life carrying that scar. Some won't take part in card or other games, or learn to drive a car, because they believe they are inferior and are fearful of being shown up as such. If someone of Mr Benson's calibre could ask me to treat him like an idiot, then who was I to pretend I had an answer for everything?

My encounter with Mr Benson had the effect of opening a window on knowledge. How wonderful not to have to pretend you are bright. As you accumulate knowledge, so you gain confidence and eventually realize that you are actually bright. But you have to be taught by someone who is capable of expressing themselves properly.

The contribution made to my enlightenment by Mr Benson just seemed to point up the futility of my existence at Peat Marwick. He wasn't a bluffer, but I would have to become one if I was to build an impressive curriculum vitae and make contact with the right people. I did not have the stomach for it, and fortunately neither did Ellen. After just one year's post-qualification experience, I turned my back on the City and started looking for a job in what I perceived to be the 'real world'.

The Real World

The option open to me was to obtain a position with a company either as Company Secretary, Accountant, Financial Controller or whatever fancy title you wished to give it. The usual course was to start off as Assistant Secretary, then after gaining the necessary experience to apply for a position in another company as the genuine article. I didn't like the idea of this because the assistants I had come across were never given responsibility. They were more stooges than assistants and consequently were not enabled to gain real experience. When the top job did become vacant – almost exclusively as a result of retirement or premature death – the stooge image prevented their promotion aspirations being taken seriously and in many cases a replacement was brought in from outside. I wanted to be the man in charge.

Eventually I accepted a position as accountant in Eustace & Partners, a small but expanding company that had reached the stage of needing a full-time accountant. I was jumping straight in at the deep end, not sure whether I would sink or swim. It was a very close call. With discretionary and appropriate use of Aungiers-isms and Bensonisms, I soon learned to keep afloat and in no time at all became a very strong swimmer.

While I was at Eustace & Partners I made my next

serious attempt to quit smoking. I decided to switch from cigarettes to a pipe. My logic was quite sound. Loathing the smell of pipe tobacco, I reasoned that I would not enjoy smoking it, would get fed up and eventually not want to smoke at all. As any pipe smoker will know, the novice not only has to get used to the foul smell but the pipe itself. The continual sucking on the stem made the tip of my tongue so sore after a few weeks that it felt as though it had a boil on it. The pipe I had chosen was one that I felt fitted my image of a modern man about town, with the stem coming out straight from a small bowl. I would have done better to have followed the example of my hero Sherlock Holmes and chosen a traditional style of pipe with downward curving stem and huge bowl. By far the worst part of pipe smoking is coping with the residual goo that collects in the bottom of the bowl, especially if, like me, you fail to clean it out regularly. One of my most embarrassing moments came after a meal at a restaurant with friends. I lit up, tilted my head back slightly to inhale the rich fumes and got a throat-load of goo. I threw up instantly.

Three months later my tongue was still sore, and I wasn't enjoying the taste of the tobacco, despite constantly experimenting with different types. But I persevered and learnt to cope with both the tobacco and the ongoing maintenance. I was smoking two ounces of Balkan Sobranie a day and after a while was also accepting 'just one' cigarette. In no time at all I had cast the pipe aside for good and reverted to smoking cigarettes.

Given my frequent failed attempts to stop smoking, I reached the point where I thought quitting entirely was out of the question. Cutting down had to be the next best option. I decided to restrict myself to ten a day.

Initially this worked well. Each hour of every day, I had a little reward to look forward to. Soon I became a permanent clock-watcher, noting each minute of my life as it ticked away. I was meticulously strict, never allowing myself to light up before the minute hand had reached the hour. Occasionally I would stand there, cigarette in mouth, waiting for the second hand to reach the vertical. What a state I got into, exercising the willpower and self-discipline it required to stick to my regime. It took about ten minutes to smoke that precious cigarette. Once it was finished, I had to wait fifty minutes for the next one. Eventually I had one of those days when everything that could go wrong did. I could no longer restrict myself. No problem, I told myself, I'll start again tomorrow.

The Irish comedian Dave Allen has summed up very accurately what can happen when you try to control your nicotine intake:

'I have a very strict rule about smoking. I never smoke more than an average of ten cigarettes a day. Occasionally I might borrow the odd cigarette from the next day's quota, but I never, ever exceed the average of ten a day. The cigarette that I am now smoking is part of my quota for the fourth of July two thousand and forty-six!'

I didn't fall into this particular trap. In fact, I did the complete opposite. When the hour was up, instead of lighting the cigarette, I would go the whole of the next hour without one. Sometimes I would smoke only one or two cigarettes throughout the whole day. I was like a squirrel burying a reserve of nuts for the winter. But it wasn't helping me to stop smoking or making cigarettes seem less precious. I remember the first time I built up ten credits. I was like an excited child counting out the pennies hoarded in its piggy-bank. I decided I would blow the lot next day. The sheer luxury of being able to smoke twenty whole cigarettes in one day was bliss!

But the day after was torture. I had to go back to the discipline of one an hour. Eventually my resistance ran out. There was no way I could survive on one cigarette an hour. I tried one cigarette every half-hour. I reasoned that twenty a day couldn't be that bad. But still the intake was not enough to prevent me thinking about cigarettes for the twenty minutes of that half-hour when I was not smoking. Wishing two-thirds of your life away is not much different from wishing five-sixths of it away. Both add up to a miserable existence. In the end I decided not to smoke during the day and to save the whole lot for when I got home. Again, it was great in the beginning. All day I would abstain and feel like a saint. On the stroke of 5.30 I would hurtle out of the office, race home and immediately light up. That first cigarette was wonderful. The next? Not quite as good. By the time I was chain-smoking the fifth cigarette, I'd be thinking:

'Why am I doing this?'

After two years as a fully qualified accountant I was brimming with confidence and felt competent enough to become financial director of ICI, not that such a position would ever have been offered to a 25-year-old in those days. But I was ready to move on again. William Cory & Sons were advertising for several assistant accountants. I still had not the slightest desire to be an assistant, but the salaries on offer were exceptionally high and Cory's was a household name. It would give my CV quite a boost to land a job there so early in my career. With nothing to lose, I applied and was invited for an interview.

Cory's head office was situated in a depressing building near Whitechapel, a 20-minute walk from Wapping. Nor was I impressed with the man who would be my boss. Midway through the interview I decided that Cory's was not for me. I was about to tell the interviewer as much, when he said, 'Cory's operate a strict no-smoking policy.' Nowadays such a policy is the rule rather than the exception, but in the early Sixties it was virtually unheard of. You would have thought his revelation would have given me, a chainsmoker, the ideal opportunity to end the interview there and then. I said nothing, and when I was offered a position, I accepted it.

Admittedly the salary was good but that wasn't the principal factor motivating me. I know of many cases where smokers have refused a job because they weren't allowed to smoke. I'm sure I'm not unique, but I'm the only person I've heard of who accepted a job he didn't want for the sole purpose of forcing himself to quit! I took that job because it seemed the right course of action. At the forefront of my mind was an experience I had had some months earlier, at the Royal Marsden Hospital.

My father was in that hospital dying of lung cancer. He was 56 years old. When I arrived at his bedside he was barely conscious and I was convinced he was not aware of my presence. He made a few guttural sounds that were unintelligible to everyone but my mother. She took a straw, dipped it in a glass of water and allowed a drop to settle on his parched lips. When the drop seeped into his mouth, he choked on it. He was a man who enjoyed his pint, so much so that he had spent every night in the pub. I had despised him for that, but at this moment I would have given anything to quench his thirst. His last words to me were to make me promise to quit smoking.

I made that promise without hesitation. I'd already

decided that no way would I end up like him. The moment I left the hospital, I lit a cigarette.

The offer of that job at Cory's seemed like a way of atoning for my betrayal as well as halting a noticeable deterioration in my own health. Since qualifying I had been able to afford the best cigarettes, and as many of them as I wanted. Their adverse effects were becoming increasingly obvious. Cory's presented me with a golden opportunity to overcome the problems I had previously encountered when attempting to quit, and to keep that promise I had made.

For some smokers the biggest hurdle is the need to smoke on social occasions. They can withstand the siren voice of nicotine while they are working, but put them in a pub, a restaurant or just relaxing with friends and they must have a cigarette. Other smokers are convinced they can't concentrate without a cigarette to draw on. I was one of those smokers. I thought that if I worked in an office where I wasn't allowed to smoke, I would have no choice but to quit. But as I would discover many years later, trying to force yourself to quit is a very common – and unsuccessful – tactic among smokers.

In those days it was thought that if somebody wanted to quit smoking, all they required was a little willpower. On the face of it I was cutting the mustard as a dynamic young accountant. Dig deeper and the truth was that I could not admit to my wife, family and friends that I didn't possess sufficient willpower to quit. The only way I thought I could succeed was to accept a job I didn't like just because it had a no-smoking policy. If you've been an alcoholic, or at the mercy of any other form of addiction, you will be familiar with the term 'denial'. For the lucky ones among you, 'denial' is basically the process by which an addict refuses to accept that they are addicted and searches for any excuse to justify their irrational actions. I was in denial.

Even now, when so much more is known about nicotine addiction, smokers will deny that they smoke because they are addicted. Most will maintain that they smoke because they choose to. Ask them when they decided to smoke their first experimental cigarette and the vast majority of them will remember the occasion, if not the date. But ask them when they decided to smoke every day for the rest of their lives and all you'll get is a blank stare.

The official office hours at Cory's were nine to five with an hour for lunch. I spent the mornings waiting for lunch and the afternoons waiting for five o'clock. If I had a particularly tricky problem, I would have crafty cigarettes in the toilet in order to solve it. In no time a rumour was going round that I suffered from dysentery.

However, much worse was to come. If you have ever watched the TV series *The Fall and Rise of Reginald Perrin* you will remember that he arrived late for work at Sunshine Desserts every morning and each day came up with some ingenious excuse. I found myself in a similar situation. I wasn't late, but the company was undergoing a substantial reorganization, and as the accountant in charge of setting up the Wharfage and Lighterage division I was expected to work overtime. By 5 o'clock I was so desperate for a cigarette that I just had to get out as soon as possible, to satisfy my craving for nicotine and calm the twitchiness that accompanied its withdrawal. I found myself continually making the promise to work late and then over-turning this with a reason not to. My seeming lack of willpower and my perception of how I must be coming over to my work colleagues sent my self-esteem plummeting. Such was the power of nicotine, my career became a poor second to my need to smoke, and I was helpless to change the situation. After six months I could stand the strain no longer and began searching for another job. I was so desperate I accepted the first position offered.

This came from a company that had been formed to market an innovative product called Autolock. The brain-child of the nephew of the man who had invented traffic lights, this device was intended to protect cars against theft by the installation of a combination lock into which you had to enter the right numbers before the engine would start. Any car fitted with Autolock was as good as burglar-proof, or so the advertising went.

Initial demand for the product had exceeded all expectations and the company was in desperate need of an accountant and office manager to restore order to their books and accounting procedures. Although making this move would involve a considerable drop in salary, the prospects were good and the directors came across as dynamic go-getters. The job was exactly what I wanted, and was made even more attractive by its proximity to my home in Putney. There was only one rather serious snag – if I wanted it, I had to start the following Monday.

I was on one month's notice with Cory's, and had I refused to give it my future prospects would have been seriously handicapped by not being able to provide a reference from them. As I couldn't offer a genuine reason for leaving the firm almost instantly, I racked my brains for a way out. Aungiers' training in office politics had come to my aid on a few occasions since leaving Peat Marwick, and it did so again. Somehow, I reasoned, Cory's had to be persuaded that it was in their interest to let me go as soon as possible.

My boss wanted me to serve out my notice, and so pressure had to be brought on him from another quarter. I had noticed at my interview a certain animosity between him and the personnel director, who seemed very dubious about the need for hiring all these extra accountants, seven in all. My boss had one as his assistant who appeared not to undertake any accountancy functions. After pointing out to my boss that my place could easily be taken by this character, I went to the personnel director and told him I wanted to leave as soon as possible because I was bored with sitting around all day twiddling my thumbs. Delighted by the prospect of saving the company money, he arranged for me to leave immediately, with an excellent reference.

Autolock was probably the only period in my life as an accountant that I enjoyed. I worked all the hours under the sun in order to establish office routines and to catch up with the back-log. There was no sliding off to the toilets to defy a smoking ban, and my co-workers were young and ambitious, much like myself. I was kept so busy sorting out the office procedures that it took longer than it would have done for me to realize the management were not all they appeared. Although the conception of the Autolock was ingenious, the application itself had not been perfected. At the press launch, a brand new Ford Zodiac saloon fitted with the device had been offered free to anybody who could start it within an hour. If someone had accepted the challenge (surprisingly, no one had), the car would not have started no matter what number had been dialled. The promoters had taken the precaution of emptying the petrol tank.

More serious was the way the operation was set up financially. Autolock was a subsidiary of a public insurance company and was financed by the parent company discounting the invoices. Invoice discounting is a very expensive method of raising money and is usually only suitable for high-risk ventures. We would prepare a list of the invoices for alarms sold and the discounting company would send us a cheque for 80 percent of the total value, less their commission. When we received payment for the invoice we had to repay the 80 percent. It was the job of our salesmen to chase up late payers. I became aware that many of these salesmen had been involved in a high profile scam run by 'entrepreneur' John Bloom, and was immediately concerned. I rang our largest debtor who confirmed that no goods had been ordered or delivered. Invoices, therefore, were being raised on sales that didn't exist. I pursued the salesman responsible and was told he had acted on the orders of the sales director. He in turn informed me that he had been following the orders of the managing director. When I tackled him it was pointed out that as I had signed the list of fraudulent invoices, I would be stupid to draw attention to the situation.

What he said was true, except that I had no idea the invoices were fraudulent. My conscience was clear. When it became obvious that he was not going to come clean about Autolock's true position, I informed the directors of the parent company. I expected to receive their gratitude, but instead was accused of being naive. I was quick to point out that it was they who had been conned, and but for me they would have lost more money. Ironically, some years later those same directors would face prosecution for the improper investment of public funds.

Autolock went into liquidation and I was out of a job. My CV did not look attractive to a prospective employer.

In essence, it read:

POST-QUALIFICATION EXPERIENCE

2 years as accountant of small, virtually unknown company.

6 months as assistant accountant with large public company.

6 months as accountant and office manager to small company that went broke.

Put yourself in the position of a company needing an accountant. I might be able to convince you face-to-face that I'm just the man you are looking for, but would you give me an interview? Initially, nobody did, and it began to rattle me. Not being wanted when you are young, ambitious and qualified, during a period of full employment when jobs and opportunities are plentiful, is a salutary experience. After six weeks of panic, I got an interview.

Life with the Lines

Lines Bros was a large public company and the biggest toy manufacturer in the world. I knew the name well, because it had appeared prominently in the portfolio of a unit trust I audited at Peat Marwick. I once asked the trust fund manager how he chose companies to invest in. He replied without hesitation:

'I base my decision on one factor only – good management. If a company has good management, it cannot fail.'

I made a point of remembering this comment. It seemed excellent advice, and still does.

Lines Bros wasn't well known beyond the city pages of the quality newspapers but most of its subsidiaries were household names. Even now Meccano, Scalextric, Hornby-Dublo, Tri-ang and Pedigree Prams conjure great nostalgia in my generation. It was to one of these subsidiaries that I was called for an interview: Pedigree Dolls. The name and nature of this company's business would have put off many would-be applicants, as would its location at the further reaches of the Northern Line, a world away from the plum areas of the City and West End, but I wasn't in a position to pick and choose. I was out of work and desperate, with three young children and a wife to keep.

My confidence was a bit rocky as I set off for Merton. Recalling that fund manager's words did not improve it. If the management was good, I told myself, no way would I get the job. This was a ridiculous attitude, but since qualifying I had only been employed by firms with bad management. Surely one with good management would take one look and show me the door. I need not have worried. Discussion of my accounting skills and professional suitability was secondary to scrutiny of my shoes. The interviewer told me how he always made a point of not only examining the toes of an applicant's shoes but of noticing whether the heels were polished. Fortunately, my drill instructor habits had persisted and the toes and heels of mine gleamed. I was offered the position and was more than happy to accept the company's terms, which included another cut in salary.

I later learnt that I had been the only applicant and that it was Lines Bros' policy to appoint the cheapest with the shiniest shoes. Good management, it seemed, was all about recognizing a bargain.

Although I still didn't like being an accountant, it was a most exciting time to be working for Pedigree Dolls. The company's products had an excellent reputation and we were about to launch a version of the accessorized dolls that were already a hit on the other side of the Atlantic, Barbie and Tammy. Like them, Sindy came equipped with a variety of outfits and accessories, and like them she seemed destined to be a big money-spinner.

Sindy was launched in 1963 with an unprecedented advertising campaign and by Christmas of that year over 200,000 dolls had been sold. Gearing production to demand is always a problem when launching a new product. In the case of Sindy, production couldn't cope with a tenth of the demand. This mis-match was exacerbated by the nature of the product. The outfits were so small it took longer to machine one of them than it did a full-size dress. In order to produce the volume at the right price, the outfits had to be made in Hong Kong, but this took some time to set up. The mums and dads who had placed orders with their local toyshop were let down, and so they started placing orders with other shops. This duplication resulted in orders being placed with Hong Kong for ten times the actual demand. Once Hong Kong got organized, shiploads of outfits arrived. The TV advertising campaign had to be prolonged to help reduce this massive over-stocking. Many of the Sindy outfits spent their lives in a warehouse where they became infested by beetles.

This all took some time to unravel. Serious doubts about the Lines Bros management began to surface soon after I joined the company. Whereas previously I had witnessed mis-management due to corruption, at Lines the mis-management was down to incompetence and ignorance. The policy was to appoint as managing directors of their subsidiaries ex-Guards officers who were casualties of the post-War defence cuts. These men looked the part and sounded it, but beneath the veneer of good manners and bonhomie there was little substance. Imagine a managing director in the mould of Terry-Thomas and you will have some idea of the type.

My first insight came when the MD asked me to sit in on a meeting with a lady who ran a small company of machinist outworkers, because he 'wasn't too strong on the financial side'. After the two of them had agreed a price for producing the outfits, the MD asked for my comments. I said to the lady, 'I presume you'll be happy with the usual 5 percent cash discount for monthly settlement?' Anyone who has been in business will know the usual rate is $2^{1/2}$ percent. Seemingly unaware that she was giving the discount and not receiving it, she said: 'Can't you make it 10 percent?' Before I could reply, the MD chipped in with: 'Let's split the difference and make it $7^{1/2}$ per cent.' Clearly, he was labouring under the same misapprehension.

Given the volumes of dolls we were planning to sell, simplicity of manufacture was integral to our success, and this was in turn dictated by the cleverness of the designs for Sindy's wardrobe. I was under the impression that the Sindy outfits were being designed by experts. At the first general progress meeting I attended, I discovered that our 'design expert' had studied dress-making at school and was none other than the MD's wife. She arrived late and harassed, explaining that the au pair was sick so she had to bring along their six-month-old baby. The baby cried throughout the meeting. When it was the turn of the 'design expert' to speak, she handed the baby over to the sales director, who continued making cooing noises over his charge even after it had been sick over his immaculate pin-striped suit.

The sales director at Pedigree was about one step ahead of the MD when it came to a grasp of figures. Asked to devise an incentive scheme to boost sales, he turned to me for help. I suggested that each salesman be given a target based on the level of sales achieved in the previous year and that he be paid a commission of 10 percent on sales achieved over and above his target. This rate of commission, we agreed, was the minimum required to create the necessary incentive. The sales director was delighted with the simplicity of the scheme and together we took it to the MD for his approval. I had agreed to let the sales director explain the scheme to the MD, and this he did very concisely and carefully. Approval should have been a formality, but once again the MD's ignorance got in the way:

MD: 'If a chap did bring in £1000 over his target, how much commission would he earn?'

SD: '10 percent.'

MD: 'How much would that be in actual cash?'

SD (*looking somewhat confused and suspecting a trick question*): 'Do you mean after making deductions for PAYE and NHI?'

MD (*somewhat curtly*): 'No, let's try to keep it as simple as possible, shall we.'

SD (*struggling with the disconcerting knowledge that the man running the business couldn't work out 10 percent of £1000*): 'Well, er, £100'.

MD (*now sounding very masterful and sure of his ground*): 'I see, I see. And if I reduce the rate to 5 per cent, what then?'

SD (*in a flat tone, having accepted that our MD has less mathematical sense than the average 8-year-old*): '£50.'

MD (*without hesitation*): 'That's settled the matter. We'll make it 5 percent.'

The MD gave the impression of being very pleased with his decision. Presumably because he thought he had saved the firm a fortune in commission. His short-sightedness resulted in not one salesman reaching the target.

I was now very concerned about the company's direction, and told Ellen I was sure the company would go broke unless there was a change at the top. She thought I was worrying unnecessarily, and reminded me that it was the biggest toy company in the world and that the management was reputed to be excellent. Neither argument gave me comfort, especially as I was now receiving almost daily reports of the MD's ineptitude from other officers in the company, from the factory director to the export sales director. The company couldn't survive long at the rate it was losing money. As I was responsible for the bottom line, I felt it was my duty to do something about our situation.

The question was how should I go about it. Although the MD was severely lacking in business acumen, he was a very nice, compassionate person and a gentleman in every sense of the word. No way could I have gone to him and suggested that he should resign because he was a complete idiot and out of his depth. On the other hand, I couldn't bring myself to go above his head; the code ingrained in me as a street urchin and latterly in the RAF said you don't snitch on a friend or colleague. Nothing in my accountancy training or previous experience remotely prepared me for the bind I was in.

Fortunately the situation resolved itself. After presenting a set of accounts that reflected the sad state of affairs, I was hauled up before the chief accountant of the parent company and asked to explain the losses. I could only do this by relating some of the ridiculous decisions made by the MD. The upshot was that he was sacked and we were merged into the Rovex division of the Lines empire which included toymakers Tri-ang, Meccano and Scalextric. I was appointed financial controller of Rovex.

It seemed appropriate to make yet another attempt to give up smoking. By this point in my smoking career, 1965, my number of failures was growing steadily. Having failed miserably with willpower methods, I had hit on a brilliant new strategy: I would stop buying cigarettes. This approach wasn't unique and it wasn't particularly successful. I didn't let either consideration deflate my enthusiasm. I would be different from all those others who had failed because I had worked out the reason for their failure: they had felt guilty about accepting 'freemans' from their friends. In my experience guilt always eventually drove the would-be quitter to buy a packet. After all, isn't this how we all get hooked in the first place? I warned friends and acquaintances in advance that I'd accept all offers of cigarettes without guilt or feeling obliged to reciprocate.

The response was staggering. People who had never previously offered me cigarettes did so. The situation was typical of all drug addiction. When you are hooked and desperately needing a fix, no one will give you one. But once other addicts sense you are trying to escape, they will do all they can to keep you in the trap. Smokers will just keep blowing smoke in your face and thrusting cigarettes at you. When this happened to me, it was marvellous at first. I got immense satisfaction from anticipating the annoyance of those many 'pushers' when I didn't get hooked again, despite the regular supply of free cigarettes.

However, human nature will out, and the once plentiful supply dried up until eventually I was down to one source, my secretary. I had typical addict's schizophrenia: half of my brain hated her for pushing the drug, while the other half loved her for being my lifeline. Guilt began to creep in after a few weeks, but I dismissed it and stuck rigidly to my plan not to buy cigarettes. My brain worked out the problem for me: buy a packet for her, it said. After three months I was buying three packets of her favourite brand every morning. I could now accept cigarettes from her with a clear conscience and still kid myself that I was stopping smoking because I did not particularly like her brand. After a few weeks I went back to buying my favourite brand for myself.

On the job front, my initial hope that the change in management structure would be for the better was quickly dashed. The MD of Rovex turned out to be another ex-Guards officer and marketing man. He used to refer to himself as an 'ideas man', which in my experience is a term for people who have never been trained to perform a useful job. One of his brilliant ideas to boost sales was ankle bands to help children learn to swim. When he unveiled this at a meeting, we thought he must be joking. He wasn't. The sales director passed him a doodle of a pair of child's feet appearing above the surface of water. The idea wasn't pursued.

As financial director I came into regular contact with the board of the parent company, and the men who were responsible for the parlous state of management in its various branches. The board was completely dominated by its chairman, who had no more idea of running a business than the people he was appointing, all of whom were 'yes' men.

At a meeting of the divisional financial directors he proclaimed: 'I want office costs to be cut by 25 percent.' The chief 'yes' man was quick to confirm that he would make sure it was done. The others eventually followed suit, if somewhat reluctantly.

CH: 'What about you Mr Carr?'

Me: 'I'm just wondering which functions we can cut out.'

CH: 'I don't want you to cut out any functions, just cut your costs by 25 percent. If the others can do it, why can't you?'

Me: 'Because I consider it part my job to keep costs to a minimum on a continual basis. If I'd asked one of my staff that question and they'd agreed, I'd want to know why they hadn't done so already.'

This response didn't exactly make me flavour of the month with the other financial directors, nor with the chairman. He didn't want to hear the truth because he didn't know how to handle it. His only course of action on such occasions was to sulk. He didn't speak to me for six months. I should have been prepared for this reaction. The first time we had a meeting at the factory, he was put out by an injury to his ego.

Pedigree Dolls was blessed with a gem of a gateman called Albert, an ex-Army sergeant. He wasn't the brightest individual but he was honest and vigilant. No one was allowed to get in or out of our gate without the correct authorization. I arrived in my office one morning to find the chairman fuming from the indignity of being denied access to his own factory. Albert had never set eyes on the chairman before, and I hadn't thought it necessary to have a picture of him hung in Albert's hut to avoid the potential for embarrassment. I was delighted. Albert was clearly doing his job properly. The chairman wanted me to sack him, and it took several minutes to persuade him of the fact that honest, capable security staff are hard to come by.

More worrying than his lack of man-management skills was his inability to grasp business fundamentals. He proclaimed that stocks were too high and sales were too low and that no more materials were to be purchased until the position had been remedied. We reached the point where purchases were nil, but sales and production were virtually the same, as was the stock level. He was apoplectic. The production director tried to explain that the bulk of the stock was obsolete. A train set consisted of over a hundred different parts and if just one vital screw could not be purchased, there was no production and consequently no sales. The sensible course would have been to reduce the price of the obsolete stock and sell it off. But that would have meant accepting the loss in the accounts and as Lines was operating on a huge unsecured overdraft from Lloyds based on an over-valuation of obsolete stock this was considered out of the question. The upshot was that the obsolete stock continued to pile up, adding to our costs.

I began to feel sorry for the chairman. On the face of it he seemed to have everything going for him. In reality he was floundering in his own ignorance, surrounded by incompetents who should have been filling the gaps in his knowledge. In a last desperate move, he resorted to bringing in management consultants. This had the effect of hastening the inevitable. The consultants introduced new procedures that increased costs but did nothing to solve the underlying problems, all of which were basically caused by bad management and failure to follow sound business principles. Although Lines Bros was a public company and accountable to its shareholders, it was still controlled and run by members of the Lines family. Turkeys, as they say, don't vote for Christmas and these people weren't going to sack themselves.

Lines rapidly fell apart and in 1971 went into voluntary liquidation. Economic conditions were blamed, but the cause of the company's decline was more fundamental. The founders of the original business, set up in 1870, G. & J. Lines, were the brothers George and Joseph Lines, with Joseph taking the leading role. Three of his four sons, William, Walter, and Arthur, set up Lines Bros Limited in 1919. Twelve years later they changed the brand name from Lines to Tri-ang, as a pun on their surname (three lines make a triangle). The three brothers were obviously competent businessmen and under their leadership the business rapidly grew. The decline started when their sons joined the firm, and over time demonstrated that they did not have their fathers' acumen nor the same enthusiasm for its wellbeing. Unfortunately, this is a very common scenario. A father spends a lifetime building a business which he hopes to hand over to his son. There is no reason why the son should have the same interest in that particular business – or indeed any business – as the father. His talents might lie in a completely different direction. It is the fault of the father if he does not recognize this reality.

In any business, if each individual concentrates on working for the success of the company, regardless of what he personally will get out of it financially, the company will be successful. When I first joined Lines I based my decisions on what was best for the company. I soon discovered that the majority of the executives, including the directors, based their decision-making on what was best for them. When it became patently obvious that, despite the best efforts of employees like myself, the company could not be saved from liquidation, I joined the 'look after No. 1 brigade' à la Brian Aungiers. In the final months of the company's life, I remember one particularly fraught board meeting where Aungier's skill at buck-passing served me particularly well. The sales director was the first target of our chairman, himself a past master at shifting responsibility. After the poor sales figures, I anticipated that the next item on his hit list would be the level of debt, which was my area of responsibility. While the sales director was still on the rack, I turned to him and said, 'What's the bad debt situation like, Ken?'

It didn't occur to anyone round that table, least of all the flustered Ken, that I was the one who should have been answering that question.

The less flattering of my friends suggested that I was somehow the cause of the company's misfortune. I had no answer for that. It is an undoubted fact that the bearer of bad news is often regarded as its architect, and at Lines I had been viewed as a Jeremiah for raising objections every time an unprofitable move was taken. The demise of Lines led me to question the advice of that trust fund manager, and wonder about the way companies are assessed. All an investor has to go on are results, but even these can be suspect when directors resort to window-dressing and deliberate distortions.

Although my career with the company ended in tears, I had no regrets. My time spent there was exciting and rewarding. If I'd taken the usual route and become an assistant accountant in a steady business, I would have been involved in maintaining existing procedures. Anyone can do that. At Lines I was engaged in aspects of business that most accountants don't experience in a lifetime. I'd been setting up efficient procedures and controls to ensure fiscal transparency, in the face of management incomprehension and resistance to change. That was a far greater challenge. More important, I had experienced at first hand the reasons for business failure. My CV was in tatters, but I was no longer worried about convincing yet another executive that I would be worth hiring. My faith in British industry and the corporate life had collapsed with the company. I decided I would never again be an employee. Never again was I going to entrust my livelihood to idiots or charlatans. If I couldn't do better than the incompetents I'd been working for, I didn't deserve to make a living.

Joyce

Looking back it is difficult to pin-point the exact time when my first marriage started to go wrong. I believe the seeds were sown when Ellen was carrying our first-born, John. Throughout the pregnancy she suffered from fluctuating blood pressure. The medical staff insisted on taking regular readings. This precautionary approach was probably intended to reassure but the effect it had on Ellen was the reverse. She became terrified of having her blood pressure taken and would be thrown into panic whatever the reading. Her fearfulness got to me so much that I began to think like her and believed she was not long for this world. When she went three weeks over the due date, I was convinced that something had gone wrong, that the baby would be still-born and I would lose Ellen as well.

The other three pregnancies followed a similar pattern. It seemed miraculous that we were blessed with four perfect babies at three-year intervals: John, Karen, Suzanne and Richard. I loved Ellen dearly but, as the pressure on me at work built up, I found her continual depressed state very difficult to cope with, especially once it became apparent to me that the problems she was experiencing were fundamentally psychological in origin. There appeared to be nothing physically wrong with her apart from the readings, and these were only taken during her pregnancies. But the bouts of depression continued even when she wasn't pregnant. My natural tendency to optimism was no match for her moods and eventually I found myself being ground down by them. Physical attraction apart, we had never had much in common or shared interests. I wanted home to be a refuge from the tensions and worries of work, somewhere with a cheerful and relaxed atmosphere. It became a place I avoided.

At weekends I was on the golf course and on week-day evenings I began to bolster myself with a pint at the local in the company of a few like-minded colleagues. Imperceptibly one pint became two. I would eventually arrive home somewhat the worse for wear to find dinner spoiled and Ellen in an even more depressed frame of mind than usual.

There is a famous Nat King Cole song with a verse that goes, 'I was walking along minding my business, when out of an orange-coloured sky – CRASH! BANG! ALACAZAM! – wonderful you came by'. The 'you' in question first came by when I was going through a very busy period as financial controller at Rovex and routinely working late. On that particular night I was completely alone, everyone else in my department having long gone, when I heard the sound of footsteps in the corridor. I glanced up as a vision in six-inch high heels sailed by. She had legs like Betty Grable, a bust like Jane Mansfield and a mass of jet-black hair piled on her head. She flashed her eyes at me as she passed and, as the man said, CRASH! BANG! ALACAZAM! It was as if I'd been struck by lightning. I was smitten.

That was my first sight of Joyce. Had she been the biggest bitch on earth, those eyes would have captivated me. She turned out to be blessed with a personality and disposition that matched her looks. After 35 years of courting, living together and marriage, that vision is still etched on my mind. No matter how time tries to erode that vision, I will always see her as I saw her then.

Joyce had been employed by sales as an evening temp to help clear a back-log of invoices from Xmas. After that first sighting, I took to having a chat with her every evening. She assures me that she had no idea of my ulterior motives and merely mistook me for the kind, considerate gentleman I was trying to be. When a permanent job fell vacant in the accounts department, she joined the staff. Having got her into the company, I was determined to get to know her better and eventually I asked her out for a drink. I told myself that our friendship would be a slight distraction, just as the other affairs had been. Both of us believed that marriage was for better or worse, and permanent.

When our relationship reached the stage where we realized we were deeply in love, we tried to end it. I was the weak link. Joyce had become the wind beneath my wings. After surviving two weeks of separation, I felt life wasn't worth living. She felt the same. We had no intention of ending our marriages or hurting our families but we were both prepared to run that risk by continuing our relationship rather than not see each other.

For several years we played our respective roles, at work and at home. Under the cover of company social events I managed to introduce Ellen to Joyce and her husband, Ray. The four of us then regularly began to meet socially, enabling Joyce and I to see more of each other in normal circumstances. Ray was a very likeable man and we got on well. When the writing was well and truly on the wall at Lines, we discussed alternatives to remaining in paid employment. Daily becoming more disillusioned with my life as an accountant, I was searching for a viable alternative. Ray told me of his plans to eventually start up a business in liquid damp-proofing, a new treatment which involved injecting the course into existing buildings. He was convinced of its potential, and once I examined it, so was I. With the collapse of Lines, he and I became partners in Merton Damp-Proofing, although Ray did not initially give up his job as a draughtsman. The plan was for me to build up the business to the point where it could support us both.

A few months into this new enterprise, my relationship with Joyce was discovered. I thought Ray would come after me with an axe, for betraying him, but he was more concerned that our partnership should continue. The business was taking off and he did not want to see it stall in its tracks over what he seemed to regard as a trifle. Joyce, he said, was fine and had already forgotten about me. The fact that we had agreed to sacrifice our happiness for the sake of our families did not alter the reality of our situation: I still loved Joyce dearly, and I believed her feelings for me had not changed. After a few weeks I stopped pretending that I was prepared to spend the rest of my life without her, and once again sought her out. To my eternal gratitude, I had been right about her love for me. I handed the business over to Ray, and Joyce and I left the district, to start afresh in Hayes, west London, where both my mother and sister were living.

Having already established one damp-proofing business, I was very confident about my ability to set up a second, which I called Aqua-Damp. I did not hesitate to invest in the necessary equipment, such as damp meters, high-powered heavy-duty hammer drills and a machine specially designed for the purpose of pumping damp-proofing solution into brickwork. Much of this equipment looked impressively technical but was in fact simple to operate. It is strange how something that looks complicated can persuade people of a high level of expertise, whereas the knowledge needed to wield such equipment effectively is often extremely limited.

The business went very well from the beginning, although it soon became obvious that expansion would not be possible unless we broadened our specialization to include timber treatments. This turned out to be just as simple as damp-proofing and it was not long before I felt confident in my ability to do a good job in both fields. I was as happy as a hippo wallowing in mud.

Best of all was the excitement of building the business. But I quickly discovered the drawbacks. The more successful we became, the greater the number of customers and staff and the greater the number of problems that went with them. People who have never been self-employed tend to think it must be wonderful to be your own boss and not have somebody telling you what to do. It's a fallacy. In business, the aggravation and stress come from being dependent on other people, namely your customers and staff. To be successful, you have to treat every customer as your boss, because effectively he is, and pamper your staff sufficiently to keep them.

After two years Aqua-Damp had eight branches, and I was looking round enviously at the people we were providing our services to. Most of these customers were couples who had bought rundown or derelict houses to modernize and then sell on at a large profit. It seemed a wonderful way of making a living: no customers, no staff, you could live where you wanted and start and finish work when it suited. If you wanted a day off or a week's holiday at short notice, you merely locked the house and went. I knew about wiring and plumbing and was also a dab hand at plastering. We wouldn't need to pay professionals to do the work for us. The more I thought about it the more attractive the idea seemed. The first project presented itself to me, almost unasked: a four-bedroom detached house in a very upmarket location two miles from Hampton Court Palace, going for what I thought was a ridiculously cheap price.

You can find manna in some very strange places. One morning I was searching for a piece of scrap paper and took a crumpled letter out of the waste-paper basket. I'm not even sure why I bothered to read it, but I did, and was amazed to discover that it was an offer to buy us out. I asked Joyce why she hadn't shown it to me. She said that we were doing so well she knew I wouldn't be interested.

Then I put my idea to Joyce. She was very apprehensive and worried about taking the risk. I drove her over to see my 'find', hopeful of being able to dispel her apprehensions. It had completely the opposite effect. We were looking at two different houses. I was seeing the place as it would be after we'd modernized it. Joyce was seeing it as it was: dark and dismal.

She wasn't exaggerating its condition, but I was certain it wouldn't take much to put it right. Structurally the house was very sound, and it had great character. The gloominess that Joyce complained of, caused by two large trees in the front garden, was compounded by leaded-light windows. Cutting down the trees, taming the jungle of a garden and putting a glass panel in the front door would completely transform the atmosphere. Eventually Joyce was persuaded, provided we got a good price for Aqua-Damp.

Our two buyers were a solicitor and a stockbroker who were looking for a better return on their money than could be provided by the stock market at this time, 1974. Part of the deal was that Joyce and I would stay on until Henry, the stockbroker, had grasped the essentials of the business. After a few weeks of taking him out on surveys and showing him every kind of rot and infestation imaginable, we were free to embark on our new venture.

We spent six months working on the house at Hampton. Joyce lost her apprehensions to the extent that she tried to persuade me not to sell it. Ah, women! Despite the result exceeding our expectations, we were both worried that we might not get a viable return. It's a risk working for six months and buying materials without earning a penny and not knowing whether you will make sufficient profit.

We made the mistake of asking the agent who had sold us the house to value it. He was amazed by the transformation. I was particularly pleased because the improvements were mainly cosmetic. The only actual construction work had involved knocking down the wall dividing two dingy living rooms to create a spacious lounge, and building a magnificent fireplace using some of the bricks from that wall. Our hopes soared with his enthusiasm, only to be cruelly disappointed. His valuation left us with a margin that barely covered the cost of our materials. If we accepted his asking price, it would have meant we had laboured hard for six months for a pittance.

Joyce reacted by suggesting we get another valuation.

The new agent gave an estimate that was half as much again as the first agent's and so much in excess of our highest expectations that we didn't believe it could be realistic. A third valuation came between the two.

One of the rules of success in the house-restoration business is to buy your next house before you complete your first. It is therefore important to have a reasonably clear idea of the return you can expect from your initial investment. We were in a quandary. We couldn't put the house on the market at the lower figure because that would've meant we had earned nothing. But if we pitched the asking price too high it might take months to sell, during which time we'd be earning nothing. We feared we might still be forced to accept the lowest figure.

We decided to go for the highest quote. For a couple of weeks we heard nothing. Eventually, a police inspector wanted to view. I could tell from the moment I opened the door to him that he wasn't interested in the house. A morose and lack-lustre character, he wandered around muttering to himself, pursing his lips as he pointed out petty faults that his wife wouldn't like.

The house had a magnificent secluded rear garden at the end of which was a 12-foot wire fence completely covered with various climbing plants. It was a very attractive feature. Behind it and situated in a valley 20 feet below ground level ran a railway line. Fortunately it was a spur line and carried very little traffic, only four trains a day. The police inspector couldn't find fault with the garden, but while he was looking around, suddenly he bent at the knees, put his hands over his ears and screwed up his face. Concerned, I asked him if he was all right, he said:

'Yes, it's just the noise of that train.'

I've no doubt there was a train but, as God is my judge,

neither Joyce nor I heard it.

'It's no use,' he said, 'we live on the flight path to Heathrow and the reason we're moving is that my wife can't stand the noise.'

I love sarcasm and the greater the exaggeration the more I like it. He asked me if next door was detached or a semi. I said:

'To tell you the truth, I don't know [which was a lie], but I thought you'd come to buy this house and since you are clearly not interested I'd be very much obliged if you'd leave me to my trains.' Which he duly did.

The inspector left us completely deflated. We decided that modernizing old houses wasn't quite the joy I'd anticipated and that we'd stay put and try some other business. I instructed the agent to take the house off the market. Even when told there was a couple who seemed very interested, I was adamant. Two minutes later the agent rang back to explain that the lady wouldn't take 'No' for an answer and could she have a quick word with me? Had I known this woman as I do now, I wouldn't have wasted my time trying to resist an irresistible force. A short while after putting the phone down, Shirley Barron sailed into our lounge. Clearly delighted by every feature, she declared this was the house she wanted. She need look no further.

We learnt several valuable lessons from that first sale. You might think Shirley was a bit scatter-brained and lacking in commercial acumen. You'd be wrong. She and her husband, Barry, had come to Britain after selling a successful business in Australia.

Most people when buying a house or a car tend to find faults and pretend they are not interested in order to get a reduction in the price. This was obviously the police inspector's ploy. Some people will even tell you they can only afford a certain amount. Nobody wants to sell to someone who thinks their house is a mess and isn't really interested in it or who can't afford it anyway. No way are you going to get the best possible price from such a person. The ideal buyers are people with money who believe they've found their dream home. People like the Barrons. I reasoned that I wouldn't get better buyers and reduced the asking price. When the police inspector heard that the Barrons were buying, he offered the full price, to no avail.

The house modernization game proved to be a very pleasant way of earning a living. Over five years we managed to renovate over ten shabby, rundown houses. Joyce acquired as many skills as I did, becoming an expert tiler, painter and paper-hanger. Those years were completely happy and hassle-free, and provided us with a good living. For the first time in our lives, we experienced the pleasure of creation. We didn't build the Taj Mahal, but in our own small way we got great satisfaction from converting a virtual slum into an attractive and comfortable home.

Our new way of life had only two drawbacks. Joyce was always reluctant to move into the next derelict property and once it was converted she never wanted to leave it. I appreciated her dilemma without sharing it. The second drawback was not one I could shrug off so easily.

I was 48 and not getting any younger. The work was physically demanding and it was impossible to gauge how many more years we'd be able to continue. I had a permanent cough and suffered from frequent bouts of asthma and bronchitis, all of which I put down to my advancing years. Of course, much of the time I was working in a dusty atmosphere, but that hacking cough together with the asthma and bronchitis had been with me for at least a couple of decades.

I can still see clearly, as if it were yesterday, my father as he was 60 years ago, cigarette dangling from his lips, occasionally dropping ash on the carpet, eyes watering, the veins in his head bulging as he coughed up his lungs each morning. When I asked him why he did it, he would insist that he 'enjoyed' smoking. I couldn't understand his response when it was obvious that he got no pleasure from it whatsoever. If anyone had wagered that I would be in exactly the same situation for over a third of a century, I would have gambled my lifetime's earnings and accepted any odds.

I suffered no illusions about enjoying smoking, and nor did I justify my smoking by saying that I did. However, I did genuinely believe that smoking gave me confidence, courage and helped me to concentrate. I couldn't answer the phone without a cigarette. It never occurred to me to wonder why. I didn't need to know the answer, any more than I needed to know why a light goes on at the flick of a switch. The fact is, it does. I hated being a smoker, and had made numerous attempts to quit. But whenever I tried, I felt naked and incomplete.

At Tri-ang one of my attempts to quit had foundered because I had been unable to prepare the monthly salaries without a cigarette. The moment I had tried to tackle the simple arithmetic necessary, I had panicked and been incapable of beginning the task let alone completing it. On the last day of the month, I had sat all morning, staring at the blank salary sheet, my mind equally blank. In the end it was a question of my staff not getting paid or me smoking to ensure that they would. Within ten minutes of lighting up, the job was done. On that occasion my attempt to quit had lasted almost one calendar month, and all I had succeeded in doing was proving to myself that I was incapable of concentrating without a cigarette. It is blatantly obvious to me now that the reason I didn't complete that task before it got to the critical stage was because I needed a safety net: the preparation of those salaries was my excuse for not being able to quit.

For my most recent attempt I had taken the advice of ex-smokers and kept a packet of cigarettes on me at all times, to make me feel more in control. The tactic didn't work because I needed to smoke those cigarettes. They were no good to me left in the packet. I had convinced myself I couldn't concentrate without a cigarette and so it had become a self-fulfilling prophecy. Whenever I had a mental task to perform, my immediate reaction was to want a cigarette. I survived six months of abject misery. One of the worst aspects was that my desire to smoke didn't diminish, as many ex-smokers had assured me it would. It just got worse. The attempt ended with me giving in rather than giving up. I cried like a baby because I knew that I'd never have the willpower to go through that misery again and that I was doomed to be a slave to nicotine for the rest of my life.

Far from giving me greater insight into the nicotine trap, these and other attempts undermined my confidence in my ability to quit, convincing me that I would always be a smoker because I had a basic flaw in my character. I would probably have remained of this opinion had it not been for a very telling comment about smoking made on television by Denis Norden. I was half-asleep at the time, stretched out on a settee, having just consumed my usual heavy evening meal. I heard him say:

'I woke up and my throat was like a cess-pit. I decided there and then to quit and I'm ashamed to say it was ridiculously easy. I had no withdrawal pangs, and I've never had the slightest desire to smoke since.'

I awoke the following morning with his words still on my mind. The idea of it being easy to quit smoking had never occurred to me before. All the ex-smokers I knew had said how difficult it was. I had heard of smokers who claimed they'd found it easy, but had dismissed them as either casual smokers who weren't really hooked or braggarts. It was clear that Denis had not had to use willpower to stop smoking. But the really significant point to me was that he had not had the slightest urge to smoke since quitting. I had never met an ex-smoker, casual or otherwise, who did not occasionally crave a cigarette. For the first time in my smoking life I contemplated the idea of quitting as an enjoyable escape from addiction, not as a period of misery and deprivation that had to be endured in order to 'give up' a crutch and/or pleasure.

Buoyed by Denis Norden's example, I decided to try quitting again, this time adopting his frame of mind. It worked. It really was easy, so easy that after three weeks I felt completely free.

I said to Joyce: 'I've kicked it! I think I'll celebrate with a Hamlet!'

'If you've genuinely kicked it, why do you need to celebrate with a Hamlet?'

How people who have never smoked can see the situation so clearly, I'll never know. Perhaps it is obvious to them that the addict regards the drug as some sort of lifeline, to be clung to at all costs. But I thought I knew better than Joyce and cited the example of several ex-smokers who could enjoy an occasional cigar without getting hooked again. Such is the ingenuity of the addiction trap and the power of denial. Three months later, I was chain-smoking Hamlets.

After so many failures I should have learnt that it is not possible to have just one cigarette. I suppose my mind could not accept that I could never smoke just one single cigarette for the rest of my life. I believed that smoking was just a habit, and reasoned that if I had got into it I should be able to get out of it again.

Deception becomes part of the smoker's make-up. Constant failure in any sphere of life is hard to bear. My periodic attempts to stop smoking took a toll on my morale. The failures were mounting, and I felt each one. If you live in a household of smokers, your seeming inability to stop is a relief to them. The pressure is off. I lived with one other, Joyce, who had never smoked. When I failed, I felt her disappointment. Ironically, although her disappointment was entirely for me as opposed to with me, and I clearly understood this distinction, I could not be as gentle on myself as she was.

The pain that accompanied each new failure was greater than the one before, until I reached the stage of not being able to bring myself to tell Joyce that I had failed. To save her yet another disappointment, I decided not to smoke in her company or in the company of mutual acquaintances, in case they mentioned it to Joyce

Like any form of cutting down or attempting to control your intake, this worked well to start with. I had the best of both worlds, I thought – I could still smoke and, because we mainly worked and played together, my intake was so low as not to affect my health. However, as is the case with all addictive drugs, as the body becomes immune to its effects the natural tendency is to smoke more and more. Super-human willpower and discipline are needed in order to cut down permanently.

Inevitably, my resolution crumbled, and it was not long before I was smoking again in front of friends. I fought a rear-guard action, asking them not to upset Joyce by mentioning the fact. Soon everyone except Joyce knew that I was smoking. Being a slave to a drug has many evil aspects, but for me this was the very worst. I pride myself on being an honest person, but nicotine so dominated my life that I was prepared to lie to, cheat on and embarrass the person I most respected.

Like a cancer, the deception grew as I lost the battle to limit my intake. I would send Joyce out to purchase materials that I didn't really need, usually sandpaper. The moment I heard the car start up, I would light up. I would estimate the time of her return and a quarter of an hour beforehand I would extinguish the cigarette and open the windows. This safety margin gradually reduced until I had to actually hear the car return before I would stub out the cigarette. Can you picture the pathetic creature I had become? Every time a car went by I would rush to the window to see if it was Joyce.

One day I was at the top of a ladder painting the windows at the back of the house, puffing away. I must have been daydreaming, because the first intimation I had of Joyce's return was the clip-clopping of her heels along the side passage. That brought me out of my reverie with a start. In panic I just flung the burning cigarette into our neighbour's garden. Luckily, I didn't set fire to his shrubbery.

I reached the stage where I was prepared to be deprived

of the company of someone I loved dearly – and, worse, was prepared to hurt her – just so I could remain in the clutches of something I detested.

We were in the habit of playing nine holes of golf together as soon as it became light. Joyce is not a ditherer and she is not one of those women who spends hours getting herself ready before she sets foot outside. At the slightest excuse, I would march off in a huff without her.

I wasn't really in a huff. I wanted to smoke and so had to get away from her. Once we set up home together, I ceased being a regular pub-goer. In my Jekyll and Hyde phase, Dr Jekyll would cause a row over some petty point and stomp off to the pub so that Mr Hyde could fill his lungs with cigarette smoke until closing time.

Eventually, Joyce challenged me:

'Are you going to tell me about it?'

I can remember blushing, thinking she must have found me out. Game to the last, I tried to bluff, pretending I did not know what she meant.

Her response came as a shock: 'You're carrying on, aren't you?'

She then produced as evidence the incidents where I had contrived to get her out of the way. She had no rival for my affection, I explained, just a rival for my attention – nicotine. As much as I knew I loathed nicotine, I could not do without it. Joyce was so relieved that the cause of my deception was not another woman that the truth was almost a cause for celebration.

That was her initial reaction. But as the months passed the signs of smoking's wear and tear on me became harder to ignore – for her, at any rate. She pleaded with me not to give up on trying to quit. On occasions she would mention how so-and-so had managed to quit using such-and-such a method. I closed my mind to all her suggestions. It was a mystery to her as to why an otherwise intelligent and strong-willed man could continually put himself through the misery of being a smoker. I couldn't understand it either. I knew the pain I was causing her and felt weak, selfish and insipid for not being able to alleviate it. If the situation had been reversed, I would have been desperate. I couldn't have borne to watch someone I loved slowly self-destructing and not being able to do anything about it.

Joyce's pleading was like water off a duck's back, until the morning of 15 July 1983. I was making my way to the car when a coughing fit brought on a very heavy nosebleed. Eventually the bleeding stopped. Feeling as low as I had ever been, and desperate for a cigarette, I lit up. The bleeding started again almost immediately. Joyce came out to investigate why I hadn't driven off and was confronted by a pathetic spectacle: me, sitting in the car, blood saturating the still-burning cigarette dangling from my bottom lip.

She implored me to consult the hypno-therapist who had helped a friend of ours to quit. I was very dubious. Our friend didn't seem completely cured. He had that lack-lustre appearance characteristic of smokers who are using willpower, as if they are waiting for something to happen, for some divine spark that will release them from their longing for nicotine. I was certain hypnotherapy was not the answer and that the whole exercise would be a waste of time and money. No one could kid me that I didn't need to smoke. But I agreed to go, purely to placate Joyce. I wanted to be able to say to her: 'Look, I've done what you asked, but it hasn't worked!'

I didn't set out with the deliberate intention of resisting

the hypnotherapist's influence. If he could have cured me, I would have been prepared to pretend I was a chicken or suffer any indignity he might suggest. I knew smoking was going to kill me and expected it to happen soon. This knowledge made me want to quit, but it didn't enable me to do it, any more than watching my father die of lung cancer had made me break nicotine's spell earlier.

My situation was by no means exceptional. Fifty percent of smokers reach a lower state than I did – they die as a direct result of their smoking. Fact is stranger than fiction. That day started with me a picture of abject misery. Who could have predicted that it would end up the greatest day of my life?

The Great Escape

Have you ever used one of those plastic fillers to plug gaps in wood? They come in two tubes, one of which contains a malleable putty-like substance and the other a catalyst. Add a smidgen of the catalyst to the putty-like substance, mix the two and eventually the combination sets as hard as granite.

My escape from smoking can be described in similar terms. Two distinct factors were introduced, they combined and then fused in my consciousness.

I was not aware of either when I dutifully made my way to the hypnotherapist's clinic. I had anticipated being met by an individual straight out of a Hollywood film, with bushy eyebrows, piercing eyes and a goatee beard. To my relief, what I got was a bright, earnest, clean-shaven and articulate young man. Before the therapy we had a friendly chat about smoking generally, during the course of which the smidgen was added:

'Do you realize that smoking is just nicotine addiction and if you quit for long enough you will eventually be free?'

I cannot remember another statement he made during our chat, but that smidgen – that smoking is just nicotine addiction – remained lodged in my brain.

I used to refer to myself as a nicotine addict in exactly

the same way as I would refer to myself as a golf addict. I thought of nicotine as a rather distasteful substance that stained my teeth and fingers. I had never perceived it as an addictive drug like heroin. Smoking was a habit. OK, it was proving to be a hell of a difficult one to break, but no way did I equate it with drug addiction. I had a morbid fear of that, particularly heroin addiction, and even in my mid-twenties I was never tempted to experiment, despite the availability of both soft and hard drugs and my ability to afford them. Society had conditioned me to believe that heroin was the great evil. I still perceive it in this light, although the facts tell us that it kills fewer than 300 people a year in the UK, whereas nicotine kills over 2,000 every week.

Like many smokers I couldn't understand why I smoked. The therapist's statement actually explained the reason – drug addiction. For the first time I saw myself as akin to a heroin addict, and not merely as an habitual smoker. The part of the statement that really stuck in my mind was: 'if you quit for long enough you will eventually be free.'

Even today I don't understand why I believed this statement. I'd been conditioned to accept the old chestnut 'once a smoker always a smoker'. I knew smokers who had stopped smoking for ten years but who had got hooked again and couldn't quit. And there were others who even after quitting for 20 years still missed a cigarette after a meal. My own experience of attempting to quit was that the craving for cigarettes got worse.

I had desperately wanted to succeed, but had never been confident that I could. Quitting using the willpower method had taught me that when we try to stop smoking we put ourselves in a state of limbo. We are waiting not to smoke another cigarette. The effect is we are waiting for nothing to happen. When we fail, our immediate reaction is to blame ourselves for having some inherent fault, whereas we should blame the method for being nonsensical.

Now, seeing myself in this new light, as someone addicted to a drug, I believed the goal of quitting was achievable. I didn't care how long it would take. I wasn't expecting it to be easy. On the contrary, I knew I could expect at least six months of misery and anticipated it would be a matter of years rather than months. I had about five cigarettes left in the pack and decided there and then that they would be the last I would smoke.

It seemed a bit late to be springing news of my conversion on the hypnotherapist, and so I kept quiet. The session was now pointless, but as long as he didn't become aware of this fact there would be little harm in going through with it. I was asked to close my eyes and imagine I was walking through a beautiful garden. This I did and very pleasant it was too. Then I was told my left arm would begin to feel very light, it would become lighter and lighter and eventually weightless and float in mid air. Ten minutes of cajoling didn't make it feel any lighter and my growing embarrassment for the therapist blocked out all possibility of relaxation. I seriously considered cheating just to get a result but decided against it.

Eventually he gave up and asked me to open my eyes. He decided on another tack, explaining that certain techniques worked better with some people than with others. This time he held a pencil about a foot from my nose and in a monotonous chant told me how my eyelids would gradually become heavier and heavier until I could no longer keep my eyes open. I'd never felt more awake in my life. Seeing the consternation on the young man's face as this technique went the way of the first was excruciating. I decided to bring the farce to an end as quickly as possible, and closed my eyes. It took a further fifteen minutes for him to deliver a string of platitudes about the futility of smoking. All I could think about was escaping outside for a smoke.

I lit up the moment I left the clinic and made my way home, that statement – my catalyst for quitting – still going round inside my head. Sometimes I wonder what would have happened if John, my eldest son, had not provided that second piece of vital information, the substance with which my catalyst would mingle and harden into an unbreakable resolve.

Joyce had told him that I was making another attempt to quit and he had brought over a medical handbook which contained a chapter on smoking. A smoker himself, he was purely trying to be helpful. After thanking him, I turned the conversation onto less sensitive ground. At this point I didn't want to discuss the subject or be told what I already knew.

After John left, I sat down with my remaining cigarettes and that book, and turned to the relevant chapter. I found the language incomprehensible. Clearly the book was intended for those well versed in medical-speak. I was determined to make sense of it and get something out of that chapter. I read it again and again. Gradually something very weird started to happen. If you stare at the pattern made by a hologram and allow your eyes to go out of focus, suddenly an identifiable image appears as if by magic in 3D. Blink your eyes and it disappears. As I re-read that chapter, a startling fact began to emerge.

Can you imagine spending your entire adult life studying Egyptian hieroglyphics, being absolutely fascinated by the subject but completely clueless as to their meaning, and then discovering the one clue that removes all the mystery? The startling fact I discovered was that when nicotine leaves your body it creates an empty, insecure feeling. By smoking another cigarette you replace the nicotine and get rid of that feeling, which leaves you feeling less nervous or more relaxed than you did the moment before you lit up.

For the first time I saw the situation of the smoker as it really is, like someone who wears tight shoes just to give themselves the pleasure of removing them. Smokers truly believe that smoking relaxes them, relieves boredom and aids concentration. I believed this, but no longer. Now I understood why I smoked and why every other smoker on the planet smoked – because we had all been victims of an ingenious confidence trick, perpetrated on a gigantic scale: the illusion of nicotine addiction. The mystery was revealed in an instant, just like the hologram picture, and it remained with me. It didn't disappear when I blinked. The catalyst and seed of what would become Easyway had fused in my brain.

I was certain I would never smoke again. I was a non-smoker. I'd escaped the misery and the slavery. No longer would I feel guilty, weak and ashamed. At the same time I knew that my discovery had the potential to help other smokers.

Part Two

The Easy Way

'I'm Going to Cure the World of Smoking'

When I made this statement to Joyce, she looked at me aghast, convinced that the experience with the hypno-therapist had caused me to flip my lid. Having witnessed so many of my previous unsuccessful attempts to quit, she was bound to be doubtful. The fact that I had not even extinguished my final cigarette did not exactly inspire confidence, in her, other members of my family or friends. They could not have been more sceptical if I had related a close encounter of the third kind. The less than encouraging reaction did not shake my belief in the potential of my discovery. From the moment I put together all the pieces in my personal jigsaw, I knew I had found a method of quitting that could be of benefit to other smokers. Up to that point I had no particular goal or ambition in life, other than to survive and enjoy each day.

Now I had a purpose. I felt like the man in the iron mask who, having discovered the key to his own prison, was now enabled to free the millions of other people imprisoned in iron masks.

After a few days of freedom from the 'weed', I felt uncharacteristically energetic. I had been grossly overweight for years, despite not touching food all day. Now I had a strong desire to be fit and healthy again. Joyce bought me a tracksuit and I took up jogging. When

I think about it now, I don't know how I had the nerve. I would come out of the house in my brand new sporty apparel, jog about ten paces and then collapse in a paroxysm of coughing. I was conscious of curious neighbours peeping through curtains wondering who was causing a disturbance at such an early hour. Undaunted, I persevered. I can remember my elation at managing to complete the trip round the block non-stop.

Door-to-door the distance was about 400 yards. It took me fifteen minutes and I arrived back in a state similar to that of someone who had just completed a full marathon.

About a year later, I reached the pinnacle of my jogging career when I managed to complete two half-marathons (13 plus miles) in the same week.

It would be fiction to suggest that I mulled over my destiny during those early slogs along the pavements of Petersham. That had to wait until I was at home with my wits reassembled. Then I would ponder. I knew how smokers fell into the nicotine trap. That was simple; ingenious but simple. Smokers smoke to replace the empty insecure feeling they get when nicotine leaves their body. When they light up and replace the nicotine, this feeling disappears. Because they suffer the feeling when they are not smoking, they don't relate it to the previous cigarette. And because when they light up, they immediately feel more relaxed, they believe this is due to the cigarette. It matters not one jot that the cigarette might taste foul or make them cough and splutter – that empty, insecure feeling has gone. Smokers have been brainwashed to believe that smoking gives them pleasure and/or provides a crutch. It is ironic that what smokers actually experience – and enjoy – when they light up is the relaxed state that was theirs before they became smokers.

They are getting a taste of what it is like to be a non-smoker. There was an analogy I could use that every smoker would understand: no one would wear tight shoes just to give themselves the pleasure of removing them. But smokers will light a cigarette to relieve the unpleasant feeling brought about by the previous cigarette. They don't see their situation in this way, of course. They are in the nicotine trap and that relies on brainwashing to keep them smoking.

I had a battery of compelling arguments at my disposal to counter the brainwashing. But I knew that hardened smokers would need more than reasoned argument to help them see their true situation. I had not been half as brainwashed as many smokers and yet I had been incapable of getting out of the trap for thirty years. I cast my mind back over all those failed attempts to quit and made notes of why I had failed. Then I analysed my final, and successful, attempt to quit. What had been so different about that last attempt? I had gone to a hypnotherapist. He had revealed that smoking is an addiction not merely a habit, and this piece of information had lodged in my mind. From this point on my particular brand of brainwashing had begun to unravel.

Some people, when they discovered that I had quit smoking after consulting a hypnotherapist, naturally concluded that the therapy should take more of the credit than I was prepared to give it. I knew the attempt to hypnotise me had been a farce, and that in no way could it have been responsible for turning me into a non-smoker. However, it is impossible to argue effectively from a position of ignorance, even if the people you are arguing against are your equals in ignorance. If I was to argue the case that an appeal to someone's subconscious can't rid them of a particular phobia or, as in the case of nicotine, an addiction, I would have to prove it, and to prove it I would have to know how hypnotherapy works. I began by reading every book on the subject I could find. These were not particularly illuminating, their authors seemingly more interested in dreaming up new types of gimmickry by which to serve up the basic technique. Unfortunately, many practitioners are ex-stage hypnotists who perpetuate the image of the therapist as some sort of Svengali figure. When the opportunity of attending a half-day seminar was offered, courtesy of a sympathetic doctor, I took it. I came away disappointed that the medical profession seemed as seduced by the delusion techniques associated with hypnotherapy as the stage hypnotists. I am convinced that hypnosis is a mis-used tool, and potentially dangerous in the wrong hands. I regard it as the equivalent of a hypodermic syringe. By itself it can not kill or cure, but fill it with an agent that has either of these capabilities and it can.

The one aspect of hypnotherapy I could appreciate was its usefulness as a method of relaxation. All of us are better able to absorb information when we are in a relaxed frame of mind. Give somebody a piece of information when they are in a panic or fearful and they will in all probability not even hear you, let alone absorb the implications. Most people are in a perpetual state of unquiet, preoccupied with personal worries and traumas, real or imagined. Smokers, for example, know they shouldn't be smoking. They try to block their minds to the fear of what might happen if they don't stop, at the same time telling themselves they'll tackle the issue tomorrow. Just the knowledge – even at a subconscious level – that you have unresolved conflicts creates fear and panic, and fear and panic are the enemies of constructive thinking.

I was certain that if smokers were to absorb my method of quitting, they would have to be in a receptive frame of mind. That was where hypnotherapy would play its part, initially to remove whatever problems are crowding the smoker's mind and help them to reach a state where they feel relaxed, warm and secure, and able to absorb the content of the method.

Joyce was understandably very dubious about my ability to single-handedly save the smokers of the world; she was far from convinced that I had managed to save myself. Nothing she or anyone else said could dent my enthusiasm, however. I was a man with a mission. Fortunately, by this time I was so adept at all aspects of house renovation that I could perform the various tasks on automatic pilot. While physically I was getting on with earning a living, mentally I was developing a structure for what I was now calling Easyway, a name I had chosen because it reflected precisely my experience of quitting.

The basis of Easyway has always been direct communication with smokers to dispel their illusions about cigarettes and the reasons why they smoke. Once I had assembled the arguments into a coherent presentation, I looked around for guinea pigs before launching myself on paying customers. Smokers tend to keep company with other smokers, and I was no exception. Since stopping smoking I had become a bit of a bore on the subject, and it was my friends I cajoled into letting me loose on them when I felt ready to test-run Easyway. Some of them had no intention of quitting. These reluctant recipients of my new-found wisdom felt it was they who were doing me a favour rather than the other way round. They didn't mind sitting in an armchair listening to me talking at them, but they certainly were not going to engage in the process by either agreeing with what I said or contradicting me.

They taught me an invaluable lesson: that the decision to attempt to quit has to be the smoker's. Trying to force someone to take that first step is equivalent to putting a claustrophobia sufferer into a small cupboard. Even if you manage to get them in, they will contrive to escape at the first opportunity.

However, other friends who agreed to sessions genuinely wanted to quit. Far from respectfully absorbing what I said, they would argue with me at every turn. These early informal sessions were tantamount to a training course, and to a limited extent I discovered what did work, and what didn't. This was where my honing of the method and my technique began. Even now, over 20 years after its discovery, Easyway is work in progress, continually being refined and developed to help as wide a range of smokers as possible. It's pointless just explaining that smoking is like banging your head against a brick wall in order to feel better when you stop. That was appropriate for me because I'd given smoking much thought during my life and had already dispelled most of the fallacies smokers are brainwashed into accepting. Where other smokers were concerned, I had to strip away their misconceptions.

After a few weeks I was convinced I'd found my vocation and felt ready to start taking paying customers. Joyce was reluctant to risk our thriving business, concerned that I was building a house of cards – one puff, literally, would blow it away. After much discussion we decided on a compromise. We would look for a place that was ripe for renovation and would also provide space for a clinic. The two businesses would be run in tandem until Easyway was up and running successfully. We found a rundown four-bedroom detached house in Raynes Park, south London that fitted the bill perfectly. Situated in a very pleasant cul-de-sac with more than adequate parking, it was also close to bus routes and main-line rail services. We planned to convert the downstairs lounge into a reception area and turn the main bedroom into my 'consulting' room.

It is said that quitting smoking automatically guarantees a substantial gain in weight. This is true if you use a willpower method to quit. Constantly gobbling sweets or snacking is a major weapon used by many would-be ex-smokers in the battle to take their minds off 'giving up'. With Easyway there is no feeling of loss and therefore no desire to compensate. I shed two stones in weight during the first few months after quitting smoking. After four months I also developed what I saw as a rather alarming addition: a lump in the middle of my chest. Typical Sod's law, I thought. I've spent a lifetime trying to kick smoking, I've finally succeeded, and now this. Obviously quitting had come too late. Throughout my career as a smoker I had told myself that if ever I got lung cancer, I would not allow myself to become incapacitated by it. My father had died in the renowned Royal Marsden cancer hospital, barely recognizable and helpless. If I was in pain, I'd commit suicide. If I wasn't, I'd continue to enjoy life for as long as I could.

I was far from being in pain; I felt like a young boy, albeit a boy with a secret worry. Although I said nothing, Joyce sensed something was wrong and asked me what it was. Her immediate reaction to my revelation was that I should have the lump investigated as soon as possible to put my mind at rest. But I was running ahead of her. Fixed in my mind was a diagnosis of lung cancer. I did not want a future restricted to the planning of my death. I could not bear the thought of giving up the development of Easyway for that. I was adamant that the actual illness could not have a more devastating effect than the inertia certainty would plunge me into. And if it wasn't cancer, what was there to worry about, except the worry?

Joyce knew better than to argue with me in ostrich mood. Instead, she told my brother Derek, who mentioned the suspicious addition to a doctor friend of his. The news relayed back to me was that the doctor didn't think I had lung cancer but he would be pleased to check me out at his practice in Princes Risborough. By this stage in the mini-drama I was being treated like someone who had lost the use of his faculties. Every time the phone rang the door was gently closed on me, and conversations were held in reverential whispers just out of earshot. If agreeing to an appointment would bring the family back to its irreverent self, I'd do it.

An unanswered question had stayed with me since I had quit smoking. If I were to be faced with some tragedy, would I turn to cigarettes out of desperation? I could not conceive of ever smoking, or even craving, another cigarette given the normal run of events, but what I was experiencing could hardly be described as everyday. Would this be my undoing?

The thought of a cigarette did not tempt me once during this difficult time. Quite the reverse: I was relieved that I no longer smoked or had that dependence. When we are convinced we need something – a drink, a cigarette, a shot of heroin – in order to cope, we render ourselves less able. Since quitting I was feeling so much more in control. While being terrified of hearing that I had cancer, I felt mentally strong enough to deal with what lay ahead. The worst time was after we arrived early for my appointment in Princes Risborough. I sat in the waiting room for an hour and a half with nothing to do but dwell on my conviction that I was going to hear very bad news. Still I had no desire to light a cigarette.

To my great relief, after a brief physical examination Dr Maisey told me that my addition was not a symptom of disease but perfectly normal. The lump of gristle that joins the top ribs had been obscured for so many years by fat that I'd forgotten it was meant to be there. What an embarrassment to be so ignorant of one's anatomy!

People often say that the doubt is worse than the certainty. I am not qualified to comment on the certainty of having lung cancer, or any other life-threatening disease. I would not want to experience again the fear of being told I had lung cancer. If I had viewed cigarettes differently, as 'friends' to be relied upon in times of stress, I would have fallen back into the smoking trap. But I knew my situation could not be improved by smoking. This episode was my first personal test since becoming a non-smoker. It was also a test of Easyway.

Christmas 1983 was fast approaching. I had quit for a full five months, and was ready to launch Easyway on the wider world. The plan was to place a small advertisement in the 'articles for sale' column of the local newspaper – by far the most perused part of the classifieds – and go from there. If we had few takers, we'd get on with modernizing the rest of the house. Our advertisement offered as many 45-minute sessions as a client needed to quit, all for a one-off fee of £30. Most smokers believe if they can quit for three months, they can quit permanently. If I failed, and the smokers who came to me smoked again within this period, they would get their money back. As no major capital outlay was involved, the risk was minimal.

Joyce saw the situation differently. From her perspective, it was tough for smokers to quit. She was still dubious about Easyway being the answer to every smoker's dream including, although she did not admit it at the time, my own. If the vast majority of the people who signed up for sessions with me claimed their money back, we would be in trouble. I dug my heels in. The money-back guarantee was a necessary counter-balance to the other major selling point in the advertisement: my claim of a success rate in excess of 75 percent. If I had not included the guarantee, I could have been open to a charge of the claim being made in order to perpetuate a fraud. The example of Brian Aungiers at Peat Marwick had taught me that bluff can serve a useful purpose. I was certain that if I could entice into our clinic smokers who wanted to quit I would be able to match the success rate I had already claimed. Once across the threshold they would discover that the Easyway business was based on sound Bensonian principles of honesty. Telling a white lie to get them to cross that threshold was a small price for my conscience to pay.

Our Very First Client

We timed our launch to coincide with New Year, hopeful that we would be inundated with calls from people who, as Big Ben struck twelve on the big night, had resolved to become non-smokers. We were sadly disappointed. Calls came in, but from friends and family wishing us a happy New Year. Wisdom is made slowly. Over time we learnt that the vast majority of smokers who make such a resolution break it either before they return to work or on the Monday morning of their return. Such smokers also tend to rely on their own willpower rather than seek help.

Joyce and I were like a couple of anxious fathers waiting for the birth of a first child. We were beginning to despair when a call came in from a Peter Murray enquiring about our services. After cross-questioning a very professional sounding Joyce, he booked an appointment. I was over the moon at actually having a customer, until Joyce remarked that he had 'sounded like Pete Murray', and that she knew for a fact that he lived just down the road in Wimbledon. For those of you too young to remember, Pete Murray is a veteran of light broadcasting who has been presenting television and radio programmes since the Fifties. If I had been presenting Easyway for just a fraction of the years he had been in broadcasting I would have considered it a feather in our cap to have such a household name as a client. I felt like a novice boxer who has just been told he will be stepping into the ring against Mike Tyson. As I went into a tailspin of apprehension, I tried to reassure myself: Murray is not an uncommon name and the man had referred to himself as Peter.

At the appointed time, Joyce and I watched through the window as the unmistakeable figure of Pete Murray came striding up our drive.

Although I had prepared well for this first session, and was pumped up with enthusiasm, it did not go as intended. I suppose it would have been the same whoever had been my first proper client. All my previous sessions had been with people I knew. There had been no pressure and little embarrassment over unscheduled slip-ups in presentation. A household name who is paying a fee for a professional service could not be expected to make the same allowances. I made none for myself and felt terrible at failing him, while making every effort to disguise my disappointment. I don't know whether he shared my perception. It was impossible to tell what he thought about the session, let alone what he had got from it. He remained affable throughout, even when at the end Joyce had to spend minutes running around our neighbours trying to get change for the £50 note he handed over as payment.

The only crumb of comfort I took from my 45-minute ordeal was that it could have been far worse. Pete Murray could have lambasted me, denounced Easyway and stormed off without paying. I was grateful that he did none of those things, and like a motorist who is severely shaken by a near-miss, I promised myself that I would sharpen up my act. Although my smoking friends had been a boon in allowing themselves to be subjects for experimentation, they had probably lulled me into a false sense of security. It had been far easier for me to tap into their particular brand of brainwashing than it would have been if they had been unknown to me personally. Until I started the sessions professionally, I did not realize how diverse the brainwashing could be.

From the time of that first session I worked on devising better analogies and anecdotes to get through to smokers. I had to prove to each and every one of them that smoking does not make meals or social occasions more enjoyable, that it does not relieve stress or boredom, or assist relaxation and concentration. I had to prove that it does the opposite of these things. In addition, I had to convince them that quitting smoking is not a case of the cure being worse than the disease, and it is not necessary to endure a period of misery while trying to quit. Most importantly, I had to prove that they weren't destined to spend the rest of their lives resisting the urge to smoke. With each session my experience grew, and with it my ability to tailor my approach to the client.

The Easyway therapy began as soon as Joyce opened the door to greet each customer. As someone who has always dreaded the forbidding atmosphere of the doctor's or dentist's surgery, I wanted our clinic to be a friendly and welcoming place where people felt able to lower their barriers. This was especially important for clients who had made several attempts to stop smoking and had failed. In most cases people tend to bring with them not just the weight of their own expectations, but also society's. Tell someone often enough that they are stupid and lacking in willpower and they will begin to accept the label. People would arrive with a sort of hang-dog expression that suggested they expected to be beaten over the head with another set of assumptions. I think they were pleasantly surprised to find this was not the case. The trend to stigmatize smokers and treat them as social pariahs is counter-productive in the overall battle to get them to stop smoking. At a personal level it just reinforces their negative self-image. Paradoxically, this was part of the brainwashing I would spend the greater part of the session trying to undo.

We started the practice of making out history cards for our clients to help us keep track of their progress. In the first year especially I was obsessed with measuring our success. At the end of each session I would enter a mark out of 100 for each client. I based my assessment on how well I thought the client had understood the method. I was never 100 per cent sure and it was a rarity for anyone to score 90. At the other end of the spectrum were the expected failures, marked at 30 and under.

At the end of the first year of Easyway, our success rate – calculated on the money-back guarantee – was 76 percent. This exceeded my greatest expectations; at the outset I would have settled for 50 percent.

The first 'thank you letter' was proof to me that we had at least one satisfied customer. Then we began receiving calls from smokers who had been recommended by past clients. It was not long before the number of recommendations was exceeding the number of smokers who had responded to the advert. Our client list was growing weekly, as was the content of our sessions, which were now lasting two hours on average. In the beginning most of our clients were local residents. But within a matter of months, smokers were arriving from all over the UK, and then from abroad. On one exceptional day, three consecutive phone calls were from smokers who were flying in from abroad: the first from South Africa, the second from Italy and the third from the USA. The next call was from an elderly lady who was terrified that I would put her into a trance from which she might never surface.

It took Joyce a full half-hour to convince her that nothing of the sort would happen and to reassure her that the session would be pleasant and relaxing. She then asked where the clinic was. Joyce told her. The woman was horrified: 'Oh, no! That's far too far!' I have no idea whether she ever made the effort to travel the two miles to see us.

In comparison with word of mouth, the advert in the local paper was not doing very well, only bringing in about one client a day. I was contemplating cancelling it, as one tiny gesture towards lightening my growing workload, when there appeared an article, written by the paper's editor, headlined 'Is he a miracle worker or a charlatan?' If he had bothered to research Easyway properly, I would have had no quarrel with him. But he took the lazy option of sensationalizing what little hard information he had to cover his basic ignorance. I didn't bother to object, but I did cancel that advert. Easyway was proving to be its own best advertisement. A few days later, we received a call from the editor to say that the paper's switchboard was being jammed with enquiries from readers wanting our telephone number. Because of this demand, he was offering to run our ad free of charge. So much for journalistic integrity. I told him that he shouldn't be dealing with a man suspected of being a charlatan let alone passing on his telephone number. I no longer wanted an advertisement in his newspaper, free or otherwise.

Joyce and I could not work out why an advert that had not been especially productive should be generating such interest since its cancellation. This phenomenon was similar to another we could not explain. Occasionally successful clients I came across subsequently would remark that they were singing the praises of Easyway to every smoker they met, and that dozens of smokers must be attending the clinic as a result of their recommendation. I would check our files and find no evidence of these recommendations.

I reached the conclusion that although most smokers want to quit smoking, it is always at some point in the future, perhaps tomorrow but never today. I am sure that many smokers had made a mental note to take advantage of that advertisement in the local paper, just as friends and acquaintances of my successful clients had probably made a mental note of the method and my name. When the advert was no longer there, panic set in. Whatever situation we are in, it is important for our peace of mind to know there is a way out and that it's within reach. Imagine you were in a room and the door to that room was locked. If you had the key and could unlock the door at any time of your choosing, you wouldn't be concerned. But how would you feel if you didn't know where the key was or who had it?

As a rule, I would ring clients a few days after the session to see how they were getting on. Often they would be glad of the opportunity to talk through points that had occurred to them since our meeting. I would encourage them to call me if they had any further thoughts they wanted to discuss. I worried most about the clients who declared very emphatically that they understood Easyway perfectly and that they were fine.

End of conversation. I suspected that they were really struggling, desperately in need of help and yet too proud or confused to admit it. However, there was nothing I could do to alter this situation. I had to accept what the person said and hope my gut feeling was wrong. Very occasionally, I was enabled to help.

After one such unsatisfactory conversation, the client's wife phoned me. She had a completely different story from his. He was nipping out to the garage with such frequency that she was sure he was having crafty smokes. Would I please ring him. Initially I was reluctant, not wishing to hassle him or risk being regarded as 'the enemy'. She told me of her fears if he did not stop smoking and begged me to try talking to him. I could not refuse her. When I got through it required very little probing for him to tell me the truth. He had only attended the clinic to appease his wife. She was the one who wanted him to stop smoking. However, Easyway had put him in a quandary. Although he had not started out with the intention of quitting, some of the things I had said during the session had made him think. Now he was in turmoil, unsure how he felt about smoking or whether he wanted to quit or not.

I said: 'The first thing is to stop worrying. You will find yourself thinking about smoking. Before long you'll lose the illusion that you actually enjoy it. Sooner or later it will become clear that you want to be free. When that moment comes, ring me to fix another appointment.'

The following morning he rang to make that appointment. It took just that extra session to enable him to quit.

Even when a person is totally committed to stopping smoking, it is not easy to reverse a lifetime's brainwashing in one session. Currently, about one in five of our clients needs two or more sessions to achieve the frame of mind that makes it easy for them to quit. Once people leave the clinic a wide range of questions or concerns might arise to bother them. Our job at Easyway is to remove any misunderstandings and leave clients feeling reassured and confident. They can have repeat sessions as many times as they wish at no additional cost, and/or phone day or night for support.

Just as I can't force smokers to attend our clinics in the first instance, so I can't force them to attend a second session or indeed to remain free of smoking after they leave. Once they walk out of the clinic door they are subjected to exactly the same influences that got them hooked on nicotine in the first place. Ironically the danger for the ex-smoker comes about six months after the session. At this distance they find it difficult to believe they were actually addicted. It is all too easy to accept a cigarette, perhaps after a few drinks at a party, or as a consequence of meeting a new friend who smokes. That one cigarette tastes awful. The alarm bells ring. They tell themselves they don't want to get hooked again. A few weeks later, when they are in the same situation of being offered a cigarette, they think:

'I didn't get hooked that last time, so there can't be any harm in having one occasionally.'

Before they realize it they are back in the trap.

Once I watched a nature film in which a large toad was shown being slowly swallowed legs first by a snake. Eventually, only part of the toad's head remained in view, and this had a contented look as though the creature had found a warm, comfortable resting place and was unaware that its legs were being digested and that the rest of its body would soon follow. This was killing by extreme stealth, a process so sinister that the prey seems in denial about its situation. Denial is one of the most insidious characteristics of nicotine addiction, indeed any kind of drug addiction. Its victims are sucked in by tiny degrees, so imperceptibly they don't realize what is happening. The sheer gradualness of the process – mental and physical – actually assists the smoker's desire not to think about their situation.

How many smokers say, 'If it started to affect my health [cough], I'd give it up [cough]'?

Our acceptance of the situation we are in with smoking is akin to getting old: the process is so gradual, we don't notice. The face we look at in the mirror each day is identical to the one we peered at the previous day. Not until we look at a photograph taken ten years earlier does the change become obvious. Similarly, the deterioration in our physical and mental health caused by smoking is so gradual that we are assisted in our desire to close our minds to it. Even when we cannot help but notice it, we tend to blame it on old age rather than smoking.

I did not appreciate the extent of the denial until I started to have sessions with clients who had had multiple by-pass operations, or fingers, toes and even arms and legs removed because they could not stop smoking. Try to imagine your doctor saying:

'Your circulation is now so bad that unless you quit, you are in serious danger of losing your toes.'

Surely no smoker would rather lose his toes than stop smoking? But the smoker might think the doctor is just bluffing to frighten him into stopping. The smoker doesn't stop, and so he loses his toes.

The doctor now says, 'You haven't stopped. Unless you do, you'll lose your feet and possibly your legs.'

By this stage the smoker knows the doctor isn't bluffing. Is it conceivable that any sane person would continue to smoke after receiving such a warning? Many people in this situation do.

The health advantages associated with stopping smoking did not register with me until after I stopped. When I was a smoker I was aware of the risk of contracting lung cancer, but managed to block my mind to it. I did not regard the regular asthma and bronchitis attacks as life threatening and, unpleasant as they were, I could cope with them. I knew little about emphysema and thought it could be no worse than the asthma. I had heard stories about smokers having limbs removed but dismissed these as gross exaggerations, merely attempts by the medical profession to frighten me and every other smoker into quitting. The permanent cough did not particularly worry me. One of its side-effects did, however, and it was perhaps because of this side-effect that I was able to block my mind to cancer and the other horrific diseases associated with smoking. The continual coughing was applying pressure to the vein running down the centre of my forehead and making it very prominent. One day, I believed, there would be an explosion in my head, and blood would begin to pour from my mouth, ears, eyes and nostrils. I managed to block my mind even to this fearful prospect – such is the power of denial.

I had always thought of lung cancer as a hit or miss affair – you were either lucky or you weren't. I accepted that my lungs were badly stained with nicotine. So what? My teeth and fingers were similarly tainted – it didn't seem to harm them. My almost permanently grey complexion I attributed to my natural colouring or to lack of exercise. It never occurred to me that it was really due to the blocking of my veins and arteries with poisons. If I had known that every muscle and organ of my body was being progressively starved of oxygen, and that my most important health defence mechanism, my immune system, was being similarly affected, I truly believe I would have quit smoking before I discovered Easyway.

Even several months after I had quit it didn't occur to me that I was already suffering from arteriosclerosis. Every night I would have this weird sensation of restlessness in my legs. I would get Joyce to massage them. It did not occur to me until at least a year after I had stopped smoking that I no longer needed the massage.

I had severe varicose veins in my calves before I quit which I did not associate with smoking. I would occasionally get violent pains in my chest, which I feared must be lung cancer but now assume to have been angina. The varicose veins gradually improved to the point where they are now almost unnoticeable. I have not had a pain in my chest since quitting.

When I was a child I would bleed profusely from cuts. This frightened me. No one explained to me that bleeding is a natural and essential part of the healing process and that the blood would clot when this process was completed. I suspected that I was a haemophiliac and feared I might bleed to death. Later in life I would sustain quite deep cuts that would hardly bleed at all, save for a browny-red gunge oozing from the wound. The colour worried me. I knew that blood was meant to be bright red. I assumed I had some sort of blood disease. The one pleasing aspect was that because of the consistency I no longer bled profusely. Not until after I quit did I discover that smoking coagulates the blood and that the brownish colour is due to lack of oxygen. When I think of my poor heart trying to pump that sludge around narrowing blood vessels, day in and day out, without missing a single beat, I am filled with horror.

I had liver spots on my hands in my forties. In case you don't know, liver spots are those brown or white spots that appear on the face and hands of very old people. I tried to ignore them, assuming that they were due to early senility brought on by my hectic life style. It was about two years after I had quit that a smoker at the Raynes Park clinic remarked that when he had stopped previously, his liver spots disappeared. I had forgotten about mine. To my amazement, they too had disappeared.

For as long as I can remember, spots would flash in front of my eyes whenever I stood up too quickly, particularly from a hot bath. The dizziness was so severe I thought I was about to blackout. I never related this to smoking. I was convinced it was quite normal. Again, it was not until about two years after I quit that it dawned on me that the sensation was no longer occurring.

There are two other advantages on the health side that never occurred to me until I stopped smoking. One was that I used to have a repetitive nightmare about being chased. I attributed this to the insecure feeling resulting from my body being deprived of nicotine during the night. Now the only nightmare is when, occasionally, I dream I am smoking again. This is quite a common anxiety dream among ex-smokers. I did not worry that I might be subconsciously pining for a cigarette. I was just so relieved to wake up and discover that it had only been a dream. I was still a non-smoker.

When I described being chased every night in a dream,

I originally typed 'chaste'. Perhaps this was just a Freudian slip, but it does give me a convenient lead into the second advantage. At clinics, when covering the effect that smoking has on concentration, I would sometimes ask:

'Which organ in your body has the greatest need of a good supply of blood?'

The stupid grins I would get in response, usually from the men, would indicate they had missed the point entirely. However, in one sense, they were absolutely right. Being somewhat shy, I find the subject rather embarrassing, and I have no intention of going into detail about the adverse effect that smoking had on my own sexual activity and enjoyment, or that of other ex-smokers with whom I have discussed the subject. Not until after I stopped smoking did I realize how far my libido had plummeted and the true reason for its decline, which previously I had conveniently attributed to advancing years.

However, you will be aware that the first rule of nature is survival, and that the second rule is survival of the species, or reproduction. In the animal kingdom nature ensures that reproduction does not take place unless the partners feel physically healthy and know that they have secured a safe home, territory, supply of food and a suitable mate. Man's ingenuity has enabled him to bend these rules somewhat. I know for a fact that smoking can lead to impotence, and that a fit and healthy person enjoys sex much more and much more often.

Smokers are fooled into believing they get all sorts of benefits from nicotine, whereas in reality nicotine imperceptibly and systematically dissipates every benefit nature has given us. I was shocked when I heard my father say that he had no wish to live to be fifty. Some 20 years later I would have exactly the same lack of *joie de vivre*. We are seduced into believing that nicotine removes or at least helps us cope with all types of fears. In fact it replaces every positive our body possesses with a negative and in the end leaves us fearful of living.

Any good therapist – in whatever branch of therapy – is able to empathize with his patients. My earlier experiences in life had taught me never to take people at face value. Each story I heard during the sessions was different and yet the same. As a former smoker, it was possible for me to enable clients to see their situation in its true perspective without being judgmental or placing the onus for failure on them. Most importantly, I never insulted their intelligence by telling them what they already knew: that smoking was slowly but surely killing them. Once smokers understand the nicotine trap, they no longer have a need – or indeed a reason – to deny the black side of smoking. Then the health and financial implications, the slavery, the self-hatred and the anti-social aspects of their addiction become powerful incentives to help them achieve their cherished goal of quitting.

Too Much of a Good Thing

To see smokers arrive at the clinic in an obvious state of panic, sometimes in tears. To see them sit arms folded across their chest, knowing that I have helped other people, but convinced that no way will I be able to help them. To observe them unfold their arms, begin to relax and lean forward to take in every word as it gradually dawns on them that they aren't hearing the usual idiotic platitudes and that Easyway is truly something special. Finally, to watch them leave a few hours later already happy non-smokers, some still crying but this time with tears of pleasure. It is immensely rewarding to be able to bring people to this point of self-realization, and to know that the process is ongoing with each new client. It is also immensely pleasurable to be made aware of how much the help I give means to the people receiving it.

However, every job has its down side, and Easyway is no exception. One of the characteristics of the method is that clients are allowed to smoke during the session, until the time is right for them to smoke their final cigarette. There are very good reasons for this. In reality smoking impedes both relaxation and concentration, but we are not able to explain this to the smoker until later in the session. To ask a smoker to abstain in the meantime would be like asking someone to dive in at the deep end of a pool before you have taught him to swim. There are also facts about smoking that smokers can only learn before they extinguish their final cigarette. For example, many smokers genuinely believe they enjoy the taste of cigarettes. Merely asking them how often they eat a cigarette won't convince them that taste has nothing to do with their addiction to smoking.

This policy was the downside. For eight hours a day, often seven days a week, I would sit in an atmosphere that was every bit as polluted as the one I had generated myself before I quit. I might just as well have been smoking again for the negative effect this was having on my energy levels and breathing. Having avoided lung cancer while I chain-smoked, the last scenario I wanted was to succumb through passive smoking, although I was prepared to take the risk. I could see no alternative to being left feeling physically and mentally exhausted at the end of each working day. Changing the method was out of the question. On fine evenings I would go into the garden, fill my lungs with air and reflect. At one time in my life I had congested my lungs to help me cope with a job I hated. Now I was congesting my lungs in order to do a job I loved.

One of the worries of ex-smokers is that the whiff of cigarette smoke will lure them back into the nicotine trap. Indeed other stop-smoking methods actively encourage smokers who are attempting to quit not to put themselves in the path of temptation by venturing into places where cigarettes are being 'consumed'. Smokers who have not yet quit often ask me how I managed not to succumb again, given my constant exposure to nicotine. Far from making me think I was missing out, the perpetually thick air in the therapy room confirmed my belief in the futility of smoking and its sheer destructive power.

More pressing than fears about the unhealthy conditions in which I was working was the concern that I was not managing to keep pace with the demand for sessions. An obvious solution to the increasing work-load was to conduct group sessions, but past experience made me reluctant to do this. On the few occasions I had agreed to give sessions to couples who insisted on being treated together, the success rate had plummeted. I had assumed the reason was that neither person had received individual attention, and drew the conclusion that the concept of killing two birds with one stone could not be extended to Easyway.

Another possibility was to train an assistant. Joyce was adamant that our success was due to my personal charisma. I didn't exactly share her partiality, but even now I believe I can do most things better than the next person. After lengthy discussions I accepted her argument that taking on somebody else would inevitably lead to a lowering of standards. I could not bear the thought of Easyway becoming discredited. With our two alternatives comprehensively ruled out, we decided to soldier on as we were.

A way of ameliorating the situation appeared to present itself after I was consulted by what I would acknowledge as a worst-case scenario smoker. Even now, after 20 years of Easyway, I have yet to meet a smoker in as bad a state as Fred (not his real name), although he had not lost a limb, a lung or been under the knife for major heart surgery. At one time a physical fitness fanatic, now he looked more dead than alive. Fred had reached what I call the critical point, when a drug addict can no longer physically cope with the level at which he needs to consume the drug to which he is addicted. Fred was using all his considerable willpower to restrict himself to just five cigarettes a day. He was long past the stage that all drug addicts eventually reach of both wanting to smoke more than he was smoking and less. He reminded me of the pitiful figure who had sat in his car on the morning of what I call the great escape.

I knew from my own experience, and that of countless other smokers, that kicking smoking cannot be achieved by cutting down. Just as the longer you go without food the greater is your appetite and consequently the more intense the experience when eventually you relieve the hunger, so the longer the smoker goes without a cigarette the more precious that cigarette will seem when eventually he relieves the craving.

Fred's nerves were so shot that I couldn't get him relaxed enough to listen to what I was saying, let alone absorb the content. At one of the several sessions Fred had with me, I thought I'd got through to him. The fear left his face, and he actually smiled, as if the penny had finally dropped. A few moments later the smile disappeared and the fearful look came back.

At times I am haunted by the expression on that man's face. Imagine seeing a child falling overboard. You manage to grab a piece of its clothing, but your grip is tenuous. You can't decide whether to risk trying for a firmer grip or just to hang on and hope for the best. While you dither, the child slips from your grasp and disappears, never to be reclaimed. I am convinced Fred slipped through the Easyway net. I never saw him again or heard what happened to him, but given his mental and physical state I am sure he could not have survived long.

When I talked about Fred and similar tragic cases to friends, they would try to console me with the sort of well-meaning phrases all of us trot out: 'You can only do your best' or 'Just think of all the lives you have saved'. I would repeat these sentiments to myself, but I could never dispel the doubt. Always I would be left with the thought that if I had done better another smoker might have been saved. The only way I could think of doing better was by making Easyway available in a form that could be consulted whenever smokers wanted to use it, and on their terms.

At the clinics we encourage smokers needing further help to ring us any time, day or night. The Easyway contract also includes offering as many extra consultations as required with no extra charge. But there will always be clients who, for whatever reason, won't grasp these offers of help. These people are the ones who are most likely to regard unsolicited calls to check up on their progress as an intrusion. I came to the conclusion that if I wrote the method down, Fred and smokers like him could read it at their leisure as many times as they wanted until they understood it.

I telephoned the most famous publishing firm I knew of and explained the method to them. They asked me to forward the manuscript. I explained that I hadn't yet written the book and had no intention of doing so until I had a publisher. They had been selected by me to have the honour of being that publisher. How, I was asked, could they possibly agree to publish a book without first reading it? By this point the two people holding the conversation were equally convinced they were talking to an imbecile. I explained that I wasn't writing a novel. My method was already tried and tested and would enable any smoker to quit immediately and permanently. The book of the method was bound to be a best-seller. How naive could I have been?

Knowing what I know now, I'm surprised the person at the other end of the line didn't hang up. I was granted an interview, however. This turned out to be a complete waste of my time and presumably that of the fourteen other people present. Eventually I was sent a letter informing me that there were already hundreds of books on the market purporting to help smokers to quit. My first reaction was to write back to explain that every one of those books was based on telling smokers what they already knew: that smoking is a filthy, disgusting habit that costs them a fortune and ruins their health.

I thought better of it, reasoning that as it hadn't yet dawned on the so-called experts that it's a waste of time telling smokers they shouldn't smoke, no way is a committee of fourteen publishers going to understand the difference between those other books and Easyway. I considered approaching another publisher, then remembered reading about how difficult it is to get a book published, particularly a first book. I decided to arrange to have 3,000 copies printed privately.

But first I had to write it. This was in the days before PCs were the norm and as I couldn't use a typewriter efficiently I had to enlist help. For six weeks I used the few hours left at the end of each day for writing. My pages of long hand were then passed to Joyce's daughter Madeleine, who typed them up. That first book was undoubtedly the most spontaneous of all the Easyway titles that were to follow. I knew exactly what I wanted to get across and how best to present it to an audience of distant learners.

Writing *The Easyway to Stop Smoking* provided me with an opportunity to investigate a general complaint we were hearing from some clients. My own experience told me that the physical withdrawal pangs from nicotine are almost imperceptible. But these clients were complaining of severe physical pain. I began to question my memory. Any rugby player will tell you that it's only after a match that he becomes aware of the scratches and bruises he's sustained in the course of the game. Did I really go overnight from smoking one hundred Peter Stuyvesant a day to zero without suffering any physical withdrawal pains, or was I so delighted to be free that I wasn't conscious of them?

The only way to discover the truth was deliberately to get myself hooked again, then quit and see if there were any physical withdrawal pains. Even though I didn't understand Easyway completely when I first discovered it, I was convinced before I extinguished my final cigarette that I was already a non-smoker and would remain one permanently. It should have come as no surprise when I failed to fall back into the trap. After a month I was up to twenty a day, but smoking them was taking a considerable effort. I had no desire to smoke. No matter how long I persisted, I could never get hooked again.

This experiment opened my eyes to the central role played by illusion in nicotine addiction. For nearly two years I'd been impressing upon clients that even one puff on a cigarette could hook them, let alone one whole cigarette. It's not withdrawal from nicotine that hooks a smoker, but the illusion that they need to smoke. Like any confidence trick, once you have seen through it, you cannot fall for it again. If you are a non-smoker or an ex-smoker, please don't test this out. You have absolutely nothing to gain and so much to lose. But you can try this experiment.

Dig your nails hard into your arm or leg. You'll agree that although you can inflict considerable pain on yourself by doing this, you won't be stressed by it. This is because you are in control, know the cause of your discomfort and can remove that cause whenever you choose. Now assume the same level of pain were suddenly to occur in your head or chest without you knowing the cause. After a few moments you would be under considerable stress.

Smokers make the assumption that the pain they suffer when they stop smoking is due to nicotine withdrawal. In fact, their pain is entirely psychological, caused by wanting a cigarette because they believe it will give them genuine pleasure or provide a crutch. Once they realize that cigarettes are the cause of their stress and not its remedy, they can no more believe in their need to smoke than they can kid themselves the earth is flat.

When our 3000 copies of *Easyway* arrived, we were so busy running the clinic that we had no time for promotion, other than having the book on display in the waiting room. After a year, we'd only sold about a hundred copies. I suppose it was a reflection of the success of the sessions. Once clients regarded themselves as non-smokers, they had no need to invest in a book of the method. It was a bit like trying to sell condoms to celibate monks. I could see no way of getting the book out to smokers who were beyond my reach. As so often in my life, serendipity took a hand.

One of the first celebrities to book an Easyway session was the actor Patrick Cargill. A few weeks later, during an interview for a local radio station in Brighton, he mentioned our session and how impressed he had been with the method. On the strength of this, the producer of the same show invited me for an interview. Thinking this would be an excellent opportunity to unload more copies of the book, I asked an old friend – who was also a first-rate salesman – to approach the biggest bookshop in Brighton. They agreed to take some copies in anticipation of the interest the interview would generate. A girl called Sharon, who had tried everything to quit, heard my interview and bought a copy. She too became an advocate after reading *Easy Way*, and did me an immense service by sending a copy of the book to Derek Jameson. A former editor of several of the UK's leading tabloids, Jameson had carved out a very successful second career for himself in broadcasting. His no-nonsense, down to earth approach to life had won a large following for his breakfast show on BBC Radio 2.

One morning shortly before Christmas 1984 Joyce took a call from one of his researchers. We were told that Derek had made several attempts to quit smoking but with little success, until he received that copy of *Easy Way* and read it. He hadn't smoked since, some six weeks previously. Would I like to be interviewed on his programme? Naturally, I was delighted, glimpsing an opportunity to get wider exposure for Easyway.

I went into the studio with nerves jangling at the prospect of giving a live interview to a nationwide audience. Fortunately the nerves soon dispersed to leave me ready for whatever question Derek decided to throw at me. Imagine my surprise when no sooner had we hit the airwaves than he waded in with:

'I hate you, I hate you! This man has forced me to give up smoking.'

I could have throttled him. In my quest to rid the world

of smoking, this was my first big breakthrough. I had the opportunity to convince 4 million listeners that the traditional methods which smokers use to quit actually make it harder if not impossible for them to do so. But here was Derek Jameson, who was genuinely grateful to Easyway and trying to be my champion, undermining the whole concept in his opening statement. If the fear of contracting lung cancer, emphysema, arteriosclerosis and other killer diseases cannot force smokers to quit, and if smokers cannot force themselves to quit, what chance is there of a book written by a former accountant succeeding in forcing them to quit?

I spent the rest of the interview trying to reverse the spin Derek had put on the method, but deep down I feared the damage had already been done. At the end, while I sat there gloomily, Derek signed off with a cheery and unexpected plug:

'I'm not supposed to advertise, but, it's a good cause. Send a £5 cheque or postal order and you'll receive a copy of the book by return of post.'

All credit to him for being a law unto himself and ignoring the BBC's strict no-advertising policy. The prospect of disposing of a few more copies of Easyway went a small way towards softening my disappointment with the interview.

I used to love Christmas as a child. Although my parents were not well off, a mere stocking was never sufficient to contain all my presents. When I woke on Christmas morning, I would find a pillow-case stuffed full with goodies. In my wildest dreams as an adult I couldn't imagine a Christmas that could equal those occasions for excitement.

On the morning after the Jameson show, we waited for

the postman, more out of curiosity than expectation that he would bring anything out of the ordinary. In fact, he didn't bring anything at all. Although we didn't realize it as we watched him saunter past our gate, it was the quiet before the storm. At about 11 o'clock the front door bell rang. Outside was a bright red post office van, and on our doorstep lolled three large, fat mailbags.

Joyce and I could not have been more excited if I had met her perfectly timed cross to head in England's winning goal against Brazil in a World Cup final. We had blown £3,000 on printing a book that had sold barely 100 copies in a year. Then, out of the blue, £25,000-worth of orders land on our doorstep in a single day. The volume of mail was maintained over the next three days. Between batches of orders we would find the odd Christmas card. I joked to Joyce, 'Tell our friends that if they must send seasonal greetings, would they please enclose a fiver with them!'

In hindsight, and looked at in purely commercial terms, what better claim could Derek have made for Easyway than: 'This man has forced me to give up smoking.'

Isn't this what all smokers are looking for – a method that will force them to stop, whether they like it or not? The thousands of letters we received confirmed Derek Jameson's view.

That interview had two unforeseen and important consequences for our development. A director of Penguin Books heard it and asked me to send her a few copies of the book. She conducted a mini-experiment by handing them out to members of her staff who wanted to quit smoking. The results persuaded her to negotiate with us to take over the printing and distribution of the book. *The Easyway to Stop Smoking* first appeared in a Penguin cover in 1985, since when it has become a best-seller in several countries and notched up over two million sales in the English-language version. Fred inspired me to write that first book. If there is a life hereafter and he is able to tune in to our dimension from time to time, I hope he is aware that he has been indirectly responsible for helping countless numbers of smokers to quit.

The second consequence of the Jameson interview was more of a mixed blessing. An avalanche of bookings hit us. I was already working flat out and not managing to keep pace with existing demand. Much as I wanted to avoid them, I had no choice but to look again at the idea of holding group sessions. Somehow I had to make them work as well as the individual clinics. This was my next big challenge.

Group Sessions

Logically it should be easier for two or more people to quit together than individually. As with mountaineers, if one slips the others will support him. But given my earlier experience of sessions with two people, I had my doubts. One of the two would usually crack and adversely affect the confidence of the other. It would be a disaster if in a larger group just one person managed to put the rest of them off. However, a far greater consideration encouraged me to take the risk. My aim from the outset was to help as many smokers as possible. A three-month waiting list was a compliment to Easyway, but to my way of thinking it was threatening to undermine our success. I was failing people by not being able to accommodate them within a reasonable time-frame. I don't know about you, but if I've made up my mind that I want to do something, there is nothing more off-putting than being told that I can't until some point in the future. The way we were going the backlog could only get worse. Three months was at the outer limit of acceptability. I had to reduce it. As far as the content of the sessions went, it was up to me to devise a formula that would satisfy the requirements of everybody in the group and ensure that no one felt left out or unable to express his fears and anxieties.

We decided to set an upper limit of 11 for each session. I was content to allow the length of the sessions to remain fluid. The individual sessions had started out at about 45 minutes, and then gradually expanded as I developed the method and introduced additional lines of argument that I felt might make the difference between success or failure. I applied the same logic to the group sessions. At the outset these lasted about two hours, and over time increased to their present duration of four hours.

I was always very conscious of the importance of not boring people. Once people are bored, they switch off and their attention starts to wander. Obviously, no one came to be entertained. They wanted help to free themselves of a terrible problem. But I tried to ensure that their experience of Easyway was pleasant and engaging. Although quitting smoking is a very serious business, there is nothing like humour to relax people and put them in the frame of mind where they listen to what I am saying and also absorb the message. Joyce would begin the process by getting people talking to each other in the waiting room. Camaraderie soon built up as individuals became aware that the other members of the group were just as terrified as they were. Joyce, a life-long non-smoker, could never understand why often the nervous bunch she had tried to relax would be convulsed with laughter a few minutes later, and as they left would sometimes swap telephone numbers and promise to hold an annual reunion. I used the after-dinner speaker's knack of getting people on my side and involved.

Most of my clients were attending the clinic because they knew they had a serious problem with smoking and had failed to quit using other methods. For many of them it was a relief to find that they would be allowed to continue to smoke throughout the session. I wanted them to smoke if it meant they would take in what I was saying. When I was a smoker, I believed I couldn't concentrate without a cigarette.

Easyway works because it strips away layers of brainwashing. However, in order for this to happen, clients must approach the session with an open mind. Even the presence of a cigarette between their fingers did not enable some clients to do this. Sometimes after a session, a smoker would say:

'I already knew everything you've told me!'

Me: 'So why were you still smoking when you came to the clinic?'

'Because smoking's a habit and it's difficult to break.'

A killer blow when I have just spent four hours explaining, among other things, that habits are easy to break and that smoking is not just habit but addiction to nicotine. Effective communication is always a two-way process.

The introduction of group sessions gave us the opportunity to re-assess an important practical aspect of our operation. For the one-to-one sessions clients had been seated in a large, comfortable armchair throughout. For the groups we invested in a range of reclining loungers which allowed people to be seated upright for most of the session and then gently lowered into a horizontal position for the hypnotherapy stage.

If my success rate was noticeably lower with just two people because of lack of individual attention, logic said it should have been substantially lower with 11. Much to my considerable relief, this turned out not to be the case. My success rate continued to rise as my experience and expertise increased. Obviously, I had mis-identified the cause of the problem with those original ad hoc group sessions.

I felt a bit like the man who had trained his pet spider, Spartacus, to come to him on command. All was well until Spartacus was prevented from responding by a malicious child who removed his legs. On investigating his non-appearance the owner concluded that the spider must have lost his hearing as a result of losing his legs.

The true reason for those disappointing early results lay in the attitude of one of the participating smokers. This person had no intention of quitting, and had been persuaded to attend the clinic only to keep a close friend or relative company. At the outset this person probably had every intention of cooperating and being supportive, but whereas the friend had actually made the decision to quit, and wanted to do it now, the supporter was only going through the motions.

The friend would be using Easyway and heading for success. The supporter would be using willpower, and still craving cigarettes. In this frame of mind the odds on anyone quitting successfully are less than one in ten. As the craving increases the supporter gradually turns into a destroyer of the friend's aspirations, with little quips like,

'We're doing so well, we deserve a little reward. Surely just one cigarette after our evening meal won't do any harm?'

Or: 'I can't face the thought of never ever being allowed another cigarette. Why don't we just smoke on special occasions?'

This situation rarely arose in the group sessions. However, it did one memorable Saturday morning, when a leading actor from the hit 'soap' *EastEnders* turned up for a session over an hour late accompanied by his wife. The couple capped this discourtesy to the rest of the group by not offering a word of apology. From this unpromising start the session deteriorated when the actor started mumbling to himself about what the hell was he doing there anyway. I had dealt with some awkward characters before but I had not come across anyone who was deliberately disruptive. I was extremely embarrassed and unsure what to do for the best. Thankfully his wife came to our rescue in true East End fashion, and in no uncertain terms told him to shut up. He obeyed and sat like a chastised schoolboy throughout the rest of the session.

This was an extreme example of a pre-existing relationship undermining the method. Generally the people who attended sessions were complete strangers, were at the clinic on their own account and wanted to leave as non-smokers. I got the impression that she wanted to quit and that he had been dragged along against his will. It would have been truly miraculous if either of them had succeeded in quitting, given the circumstances. I can report with some confidence that no such miracle occurred. Two days later his cheque bounced.

I have heard it argued that a group of smokers using a willpower method get some comfort from feeling miserable together. This is one of the classic scare stories about quitting smoking. Quit and you'll be bad tempered and miserable for the rest of your life, wrestling with the desire to light up. The relief on smokers' faces when I tell them the beautiful truth about Easyway. That it doesn't require a shred of willpower. That it will help them to acquire the marvellous positive gains that come out of quitting. Nothing is given up. There is no loss to come to terms with. In the eyes of friends, colleagues and family the Easyway disciple typically goes from would-be misery guts to super(wo)man.

When I converted the bedroom that became my therapy room at the house in Raynes Park, I designed an attractive red-brick fireplace with an integral seating space either side. One of these was the perch from where I conducted sessions. At the end of a particularly successful session, one client stood up and threw his packet of cigarettes into the fireplace with a dramatic flourish. Everybody else in the group followed suit. All of them seemed to derive great satisfaction from this gesture, as if they were finally purging themselves of an evil spirit. Before long the pile of discarded smoking paraphernalia (cigars, lighters, nicotine gum, in addition to packets of cigarettes) grew so large that I couldn't sit down without crushing objects under foot. It made quite a sight and had a profound motivating effect on clients. Not only did it confirm our reputation for being able to help smokers to quit but it enabled new clients to see their smoking in context, probably for the first time.

Smoking is not just about one cigarette or a packet of cigarettes. It is about a cumulative effect on an individual over a long period. Smokers are never told the truth about smoking: that once they start the likelihood is they are going to spend the rest of their lives smoking. If you were to show a youngster the quantity of cigarettes they would smoke in a lifetime, they would never light that first cigarette. When seasoned smokers who want to quit stare into that mountain, they see their history in it, and the futility of their future if they don't stop.

After that spontaneous reaction by one client the discarding of cigarettes became something of a ritual, and also a barometer of how well a session had gone.

Although clients were never pressured into making the gesture, I took silent note of any smokers who pocketed their cigarettes at the end. Usually those people were the ones who would need a second session.

No two sessions were identical. The mix of individuals was pot-luck. Sometimes there would be unresponsive, inhibited individuals who had to be prised out of their shells. Usually my techniques for breaking down barriers and encouraging interaction worked. In some cases, though, clients believed I could perform miracles, and behaved accordingly, as though all that was required of them was their physical presence. This was the worst scenario from my perspective, because it shifted the onus for their success entirely onto my shoulders. The 'miracle' they were hoping for could only occur if they themselves were open-minded and questioned everything I said. Despite what Derek Jameson told his radio audience, I cannot force a client to stop smoking.

As you would expect at any interactive presentation, there was a competitive element and occasionally antagonism between individuals. I learned to use even difficult situations to the advantage of Easyway. A classic example of difficulty was Harry. He was at the opposite end of the spectrum from the 'Messiah' worshippers and had come to the clinic on the recommendation of his close friend, Jack, one of our successful 'old boys'.

Harry sat bolt upright, arms folded, grim faced, silently contradicting everything I said. Twenty minutes into the session, he blurted out:

'I'm sick of this! I've had to listen to Jack for a solid three weeks, bragging about how easy it was to stop. Now we're hearing the same thing from you!'

His use of the word 'we' suggested that other members

of the group shared his viewpoint. In the early days I would have been sorely tempted to bite back in self-defence. Experience had taught me that although others in the group might agree with a dissenter like Harry, there would always be one person prepared to present a constructive counter-argument. On this occasion I sat in silence for five minutes while another client explained how Harry must have misinterpreted what I had been saying: I hadn't been bragging about how easy I had found it. On the contrary, I'd spent 30 years believing in the impossibility of quitting smoking. The method I had discovered was what made it easy for me to quit and what I believed made it easy for other smokers to quit.

Jack had not done Harry or me any favours. Pushing the method down his friend's throat before he came to the clinic had only served to identify me as a pain before Harry set eyes on me. And the pressure was also on Harry before he crossed the threshold. How could he bear to fail when his friend had succeeded? Fortunately, Harry was open-minded enough to accept the explanation offered by my defender. His whole attitude and body language changed as a result of it. His antagonism expelled in that initial outburst, he went on to succeed with the method and left the clinic as a non-smoker.

In addition to a cross-section of character types, the group sessions also embraced a wide cross-section of society. In one exceptional session I had Lord and Lady Bonham-Carter, a retired commander of the SAS, a vice-admiral, two top businessmen, and one other. The one other turned up ten minutes late, an incredibly tall, thin punk-rocker sporting a yellow and orange Mohican hair cut, a string vest and sandals. When Joyce opened the door to him, she had great difficulty not doing a Basil

Fawlty before ushering him into the room where the relaxation process was underway. This involves using first names, inviting members to remove jackets and ties, if they so wish. In fact to treat the place as home. The punk rocker took the only vacant seat, next to his Lordship, removed his footwear and curled up on the recliner.

In the thousands of group sessions I have conducted over the years, I can only remember one occasion when a man has actually done this. However, his feet were clean and so was his vest and the rest of him. Even so, I have to admit that I was somewhat embarrassed by his presence. I hope I was professional enough not to show it. I've never thought of myself as a snob. In fact I pride myself on being able to mix affably with all types of people. But I was worried about his proximity to Lord Bonham-Carter. I need not have been: the two of them got on like a house on fire, neither man appearing to be the least bit fazed by the other's presence. Both displayed impeccable breeding!

The session was very successful. I almost ruined it at one point, however. About half the content of each session is repetitive. My presentation was sufficiently polished by this stage to enable me to build certain sections to a crescendo. The entire group would be leaning forward, hanging on my every word. Occasionally on completion there would be polite applause. Normally I was so absorbed by what I was saying that my concentration was complete. On this occasion, suddenly I became aware of the group's rapt attention and their total involvement in my soliloquy. I heard a little voice inside my head say:

'I wonder if they'd be so attentive if they could see you not as Allen Carr the smoking guru but as Allen

Carr acting corporal drill instructor!'

I lost my concentration completely but managed to recover, hopefully without anyone noticing.

People came in all states of health as well as social and intellectual shapes and sizes. Clients who had to have more than one session were often the worst cases health-wise. I remember one man in the advanced stage of emphysema. He had no desire to quit and was only attending the clinic to appease his family. Every now and again he would try to have a coughing fit – the man's lungs were in such a state he couldn't actually summon the energy to cough. His face would turn purple and the veins could become so prominent I feared they would burst. On his third visit, he was in the same group as three other stubborn cases.

These other people had not yet injured their health permanently, but like the man with emphysema they were having difficulty absorbing the method. Soon after the session started the man with emphysema had a particularly bad attack. I am usually a laid back individual and able to handle most situations, even unpleasant ones, but I snapped:

'Have you any idea what you are putting your family through? Obviously you are not concerned about your own health, but you are being very selfish.'

It was a fruitless tirade and the first and only time I lost my temper with a client. The poor man was a hopeless case: miserable beyond description and yet incapable of changing his situation. Like 'Fred', whose state I described earlier, this man had sunk too low, mentally as well as physically, for me to get through to him. The other members of the group were visibly shocked by his state. One of them asked me if the man was a plant. I retorted that no one could act that degree of self-harm. The client said:

'You don't need to say another word. If that's what I'm in for, no way will I ever smoke again!'

The other two nodded in agreement. No doubt they meant it. The problem with shock treatment is that its effect soon fades. People quickly forget. They light up again and before they know it they are back in the smoking trap.

For a while the group sessions did help to relieve the workload problem, but in no time at all I was back to ten-hour days. The only respite we got was in the traditional vacation months of July and August, when any attempt to quit is put on hold because smokers believe holidays can't be enjoyed without cigarettes. In those months we would catch up with our golfing friends, on whom our now skeletal social life centred.

Before I became self-employed golf had been my great escape from the misery of everyday life. While I was on the golf course, I was like Alice in Wonderland: the real world ceased to exist. My only concerns were the slope on the green, the strength of the wind or the distance to the hole. But after the discovery of Easyway the game lost its hold on my imagination. I would turn up at the golf course and for all eighteen holes be in a deep shell of concentration, wondering how I could better help a smoker to understand a particular point. My reverie would be punctured by the occasional exasperated prompt of, 'Allen, it's your putt!'

I didn't resent these interruptions, or even being there. I appreciated that I needed the fresh air and exercise just as much as when I had been a chain-smoker, but I had lost interest in the holy grail of improving my handicap.

In my quest to help every smoker that came to the clinic, personal pride was involved every bit as much as it had been when my concentration had gone into avoiding bad shots at golf. The fact that someone's life might have been at stake was an added bonus. I became so obsessed that I turned into a non-smoking bore. I didn't become one of those holier-than-thou ex-smokers: because I had managed to quit, I expected everyone else to follow suit. I had discovered something wonderful and I wanted every smoker to enjoy the experience of my discovery. But, for our friends, my 24-hour commitment to Easyway must have been hard to bear. Thanks to Joyce I quickly learnt that you hurt people in many ways without losing their friendship, and that boring them is the one certain way of losing them. She managed to temper my enthusiasm for my vocation, at least while we were in company. However, despite repeated attempts, I never managed to rekindle my former fanaticism. My new passion was absolute, and allowed no rivals.

Losing Control

In 1988 the idea of making a video was put to me by two young filmmakers, Piers Thompson and Matt Jacomb, both of whom had quit smoking after attending Easyway sessions. They were sure there would be a market for a shortened audio-visual version of the method. I was delighted by the idea of Easyway having another string to its bow. It was agreed that I would write and present the script, Piers would direct and they would be joint-producers. The costs would be split 50:50 between the two of them and Joyce and I.

Initially it was decided to hire an expert to devise a script from the Easyway book for me to present. Unfortunately, his best effort rendered the method unrecognizable. I could not dispute his claim to expertise because I knew absolutely nothing about his craft. But if I didn't understand his 'interpretation', what chance would anyone else have? I then spent three weeks writing a script I hoped would suffice.

Two days were allowed for the shoot, which took place in a large aircraft hangar in west London. Bearing in mind that only my top half was to be filmed, it seemed a strange setting. The whole of the first morning was taken up with getting me to look right. The sweater I turned up in didn't meet with directorial approval, and so Joyce was dispatched to bring back my entire collection of woollies. When these were similarly condemned as unsuitable, Joyce had the brain-wave of calling on a golfing friend of ours, Tim Cooper, who lived just around the corner, and appropriating his vast range of exotic and expensive sweaters which she presented to our hyper-critical director. Piers rejected the lot. He then went out to a local store and bought a plain pale blue sweater. The only quarrel I had with his choice was that it was four sizes too large for me. The studio manager tried to remedy the problem by gathering the excess at the back and securing it with a huge paper clip.

Fortunately, the video camera was fitted with an auto-cue so I didn't have to memorize the script, just try to look as natural as possible while I read the words scrolling down the screen in front of me. Once I got the hang of this, we were ready to shoot in earnest.

No sooner had I started than I heard:

'Cut! Allen, I think you'd look better without your glasses.'

'I can't read the auto-cue without them.'

'No problem. We can increase the size of the words.'

But there was a problem: to enable me to see them clearly the letters had to be enlarged to the size of the top line on an optician's chart, and only three words at a time would now fit on the screen. Glasses were back on.

We started again. Almost immediately I heard –

'Cut! Allen you are moving your hands.'

'Of course I'm moving my hands. Doesn't everyone move their hands when they talk?'

'The problem is we're only shooting you from the waist up and your hands keep disappearing.'

'Does it matter? Surely people won't think they've fallen off.'

'It would be much better if you could manage not to.'

I am one of those people who naturally waves a hand or two when I make a point. This restriction increased the nerves I was trying to keep under control. I began to stumble over words. Piers cut in again:

'Just relax, Allen. You're beginning to look and sound stiff and starchy. When I came to your clinic you were brilliant!'

'My current situation is hardly conducive to relaxation! You try sitting in the middle of a giant aircraft hangar with a giant paper-clip stuck in your back and not allowed to move your hands.'

This was a low point and had it not been followed almost immediately by a break for lunch I might well have decided to end my film career there and then. After the break my delivery improved, and the rest of that day and the following morning went smoothly with none of the spluttering that had characterized my initial attempts. The script was divided into sections of about three minutes' duration. By the second day I was completing half the sections in one take and the rest in no more than three. We reached the stage of having one five-minute and two three-minute sections left to complete in ninety minutes. Easy, I thought.

I blew it right at the end of the five-minute section, and made the same mistake at exactly the same place twice more. Five minutes might not seem a long time to read without making a mistake. It is when you have been concentrating hard and intensively for almost two days. I was tired. I had a ten-minute break and tried again. Three more attempts came and went. People started glancing surreptitiously at their watches. An unknown voice came over the Tannoy system:

'Mr Carr, you're doing veeery well, but you are tending to speed up at the critical point. I want you just to relax and take your time.'

I hated the patronizing tone but I took the advice and tried again. I started slowly and was calmly determined to maintain the same speed when I came to the tricky passage. As I approached it I became aware of the increased tension on the faces of the people around me. I could sense them willing me to succeed. I lost concentration completely.

At this point everybody around me panicked. I felt strangely calm. I had faced far worse challenges than this. I blocked out the advice being thrown at me from all sides and tried to work out why I was having the problem. I looked at the sentence. It read very well on paper. I just couldn't get my tongue round the words. I suggested a slight alteration to the script and requested that on the next take everybody but the auto-cue operator and the cameraman should be out of my view. I sailed through. There were relieved cheers all round, evaporating the tension in the atmosphere. The voice on the Tannoy interrupted our banter:

'Sorry, people. We might have to do it again. We think a fly went past Allen's face.'

I was all set to laugh, thinking this must be a typical end-of-shoot joke. Then I saw the looks of consternation.

I exploded: 'This is nonsensical. Even if the fly is visible on the film, no smoker watching the video is going to be bothered. What are they going to say?: "I've just seen a bluebottle fly past Allen Carr's nose. No way am I quitting now!"'

The scene that followed would have exceeded the imagination of Lewis Carroll. A dozen grown men combed every inch of that hangar to find the offending insect. The voice ordered someone to fetch a saucer of jam. Meanwhile, one of those special lights that are the equivalent of the electric chair to a fly was turned on. A sharp crack announced that the little pest was incinerated.

What's more, he died in vain. The voice announced that it had been a false alarm. The take was fine.

Of the 25,000 smokers I treated personally, I can count on the fingers of one hand those who complained about the quality of the treatment. One or two went so far as to threaten to sue me because I refused to give them their money back. These smokers were demanding a refund after attending only one session. The sole condition of the money-back commitment is that the client must attend at least three sessions within the three-month guarantee period. Friends thought I was mad to offer any kind of guarantee; no other quit smoking method did. I pointed out that as the success rate of those other methods was less than one in ten, they would indeed have been mad to make such an offer.

I wanted to avoid accepting clients who were not sincerely committed to quitting, and had calculated that the inclusion of that proviso would sort the proverbial wheat from the chaff. Genuine clients were amply protected, if not rewarded: by attending the required number of sessions, they would get their refund and guarantee I was working for nothing. What an incentive! The clients who threatened to sue me argued that it would be futile for them to attend two more sessions. They would be subjecting themselves to more of the same, and at the finish would be just as unenlightened.

Perhaps they were impatient people by nature. Easyway can take time to sink in, and it is not a sign of ultimate failure when smokers misunderstand that first session. My attempts to persuade them to try again failed, as did their insistence on a refund. I told them I would be delighted if they did sue me. It would be excellent publicity for Easyway. Not that we needed any to generate business. We were still in the position of working at full stretch. Since we had decided to carry on as we were and not train a second therapist, all our energies were going into satisfying demand for the group sessions as efficiently as we could.

It would be interesting to speculate on how long we could have kept this up. Fate took a hand in changing our perspective one day in 1990, when I received a phone call from Richard Kalms, son of the chairman of Dixon's, the chain of electrical retailers. Richard had quit smoking through Easyway six months earlier. His opening shot was jaw-dropping:

'You should be ashamed of what you are doing!'

Although unsure of precisely what he meant by this, I assumed he was dissatisfied with Easyway. I asked him to explain why the system hadn't worked for him. Then he wrong-footed me again:

'The system is brilliant. That's why you should be ashamed.'

Before I could respond, he went on to question me about how many smokers I could expect to cure in my lifetime. I had never attempted to do the mathematics. I had no need to – it would have been a futile exercise. Clearly the number of smokers I could treat personally could only be counted in thousands – a drop in the ocean when you consider that each year about 3,500,000 smokers worldwide are dying as a direct result of nicotine addiction.

I had no defence against the point I thought Richard Kalms was making: that I should be training other people to present the method. I knew I had been guilty of playing ostrich. When I had raised with Joyce the possibility of training an assistant to help solve the problem of coping with the numbers of people who wanted Easyway sessions, she had convinced me that, good as the method was, my personal charisma was what made it work as well as it did. Close friends and family had confirmed her opinion. I had allowed myself to be flattered, although I knew in my heart that my ability to present Easyway was not unique. To argue otherwise flew in the face of logic. After all, the central point of Easyway is that anyone can quit using the method. If it's that simple, presenting it could not be that difficult.

Clearly there had to be change. My problem was letting go. From the outset Easyway had been a one-man band as far as the therapy went. I had poured myself into every aspect of it. I loved it. If we expanded there was a danger of changing the nature of Easyway. Although Easyway was a business, I had never thought of it in those terms. Easyway was me, Joyce and the method trying to help as many smokers as was humanly possible. Expansion would require me to give up my role, in effect change the way I was living. I was stuck in my mind between wanting to increase the scope of Easyway and fearing the consequences of doing just that.

A few minutes into my conversation with Richard Kalms, I had one of those surges of optimism. The sharp pricking of my conscience was accompanied by an offer of help. Perhaps this was the time for listening to fresh ideas, a chance for serendipity to rescue me again. We agreed to meet.

In person Richard was very impressive. The way forward, as he saw it, was to form a new company with the intention of developing Easyway as an intellectual asset. Talking to Richard, everything seemed possible, and suddenly the once intractable problem of expanding the clinics no longer seemed so daunting. Obviously only I could undertake this particular aspect of the development of Easyway, but his support and encouragement were important. Richard was particularly enthusiastic about the video, which had helped several of his friends to quit. He was confident that astute marketing would be the cure for its sluggish sales, and that this in turn would raise the profile of Easyway and thus assist the expansion. Although quite pleased with the final result, I had not had either the time or inclination to promote the video. I had left that to Matt and Piers, whose efforts had at least succeeded in recouping our initial outlay.

The video was, of course, one aspect of the intellectual rights the new company was being set up to exploit. Therefore, for Richard's plan to work, Piers and Matt had to become shareholders. It was agreed that each of them would receive a $12\frac{1}{2}$ percent stake. Joyce and I would have a 25 percent share, leaving Richard 50 percent. This seemed fair, because he was to be the managing director, in charge of finance, administration and marketing, and provider of the working capital. The Raynes Park partnership, owned solely by Joyce and myself, would remain a separate company.

The division of responsibilities was clear. I would concentrate on developing the clinics. Richard, Piers and Matt would jointly market the video. It seemed to me that all of us were committed to making this new venture successful in the name of all those smokers still waiting to be cured of their addiction.

Once we started thinking about expansion in earnest, Joyce and I quickly came up with the location of our second clinic. The largest city in Britain after London, only an hour and a half's drive from the capital and situated in the nation's geographical centre, Birmingham was the natural choice. However, before Easyway could start making inroads into the numbers of smokers in the West Midlands, I had to train someone to take over from me at Raynes Park.

I thought I had found the ideal replacement in Roy Sheehan, an acquaintance from Malden golf club. His qualities were obvious: a calm, pleasant disposition, good communication skills, well-developed sense of humour, and the ability to get on with all sorts of people. He had risen above a poor start in Battersea to build a career in the printing industry until redundancy had forced him into a job he clearly did not like. When I suggested that he might become an Easyway therapist, he was naturally apprehensive. He knew absolutely nothing about helping smokers to quit, or, as it happened, any profession other than printing. I talked him round, determined that once again Easyway would live up to its name.

Roy turned out to be a frustratingly slow learner. Having made the decision to start up more clinics, I wanted to get on with the job. Roy's progress, however, was bedevilled by a problem I had never experienced: lack of confidence. It was also hampered by a poor memory. I had written a manual consisting of the basic content and structure of the initial four-hour session as well as material for the second and third sessions. I expected Roy to use the manual as though it was a distant learning tool, but he proved incapable of absorbing the method from the printed page. In desperation, I recorded the manual on to audio tapes, which he found easier to learn from.

Getting Roy to the stage where I was happy to let him get on with running Raynes Park in my absence was a very uncomfortable time for both of us. I had developed the skills to make smokers see the nicotine con trick clearly, and honed them to a highly efficient level. But it had taken me years to reach that level. I could not expect perfection in such a short time, especially of someone whose experience of the smoking trap was comparatively limited. Roy, I decided, would grow into the role. If the decision had been left to Roy, I think he would have remained a perennial student of Easyway. In the end I lost patience and, ignoring his increasingly abject pleas that he was not ready to take a live session by himself, threw him in at the deep end. Against his own expectations, but certainly not mine, he coped well and eventually became an effective therapist, although I am not convinced that he ever fully understood the method; that takes first-hand knowledge of what it means to be a smoker. However, at the very least he proved that other people were capable of getting results with the system.

With Roy now 'qualified', Joyce and I turned our full attention to building a client base in Birmingham. Our plan for the expansion was to proceed slowly in stages, to finance it ourselves and to ensure that each new clinic was firmly established and making a profit before we took our next step. In Birmingham everything was in place: the premises, situated conveniently on the main Hagley–Birmingham road, the advertising to announce our arrival, as well as interviews on local radio. In my own mind I had also already earmarked someone to take over as the therapist-cum-manager: a young man called Robin Hayley.

Robin had written to me in spring 1989 after attending a group session at Raynes Park. In the letter he thanked me for helping him to quit smoking, stated how impressed he was with the method, in particular the absence of the need to use willpower, and expressed a desire to be trained as a therapist. I had got used to receiving such letters from grateful clients, and when replying would politely turn down their offer. Exceptionally in Robin's case, I did not completely dismiss the possibility, and ended my reply to his letter with:

'... if the position does change I will contact you.'

When I wrote this, I had no intimation that the situation would change. I was head down in all senses, taking group sessions and avoiding thinking about the future. Certainly, I had no intention of training other therapists. Robin's letter was no more or less impressive than the other letters I had received, except in one particular: he wondered whether the treatment could be extended to other addictions. I could not remember anyone making this observation after just one Easyway session. But what really made the difference was his persistence. When he had not received a reply after a month, he sent a second letter, in case his original had gone astray. I admire persistence, and Robin's convinced me to keep his letter on file.

Eighteen months later I received another letter from Robin, and with this one he enclosed his CV. It turned out that Robin was a friend of Piers Thompson, who had told him of our plans to expand the clinics. His CV was very impressive, revealing experience that would be pertinent to the continuing expansion of Easyway:

EDUCATION: St. Paul's and Oxford University

QUALIFICATIONS: City University Business School MBA in International Business & Export Management

OTHER SKILLS: Fluent French, solid German, simple Spanish. Communication and interpersonal skills, team leadership, computer literacy

INTERESTS: Travel, languages, journalism, psychology, cinema, theatre, sport, bridge, poker, DIY and cooking

When Joyce and I finished perusing it we observed that we should be contemplating working for him and not the other way around. Robin turned out to be every bit as good in person as he was on paper. Extremely bright and articulate, he would have no problem learning the method or dealing with the managerial aspects of the job. He accepted our offer, even though it was considerably less generous than the salary he had been earning.

In comparison with Roy, teaching Robin was simple. Although I had proved it was possible to train someone in the method without them having prior experience of it, Robin made me acknowledge that it was far easier when the person came with an understanding of how Easyway works. It is so much better when we understand from the inside out and can bring conviction born out of first-hand experience to what we do. Since Robin all Easyway therapists have been former successful clients of the method.

Birmingham was up and running very quickly, and within six months was paying its way. This would turn out to be exceedingly fortunate for Joyce and me. During those six months, I had begun to have severe misgivings about the wisdom of agreeing to Richard becoming involved in Easyway. I had been delighted to let him make the most of aspects of the business that Joyce and I considered peripheral, but it was proving to be at enormous cost. Against my advice Richard was spending a fortune on advertising the video, on PR, and on leasing expensive premises in the West End. I was relieved that the money for his campaign was not coming directly out of Easyway profits.

At various times Easyway clients with a background in marketing who could see the value of the system had given me advice. I had eagerly grabbed it with both hands and put their suggestions into practice only to find that the results were miserable. The reason, I believe, is that smokers are a very wary bunch. Over the years they have been inundated with publicity about methods that will help them to quit. Acupuncture, hypnosis, laser treatment, herbal cigarettes and pills, nicotine gum, patches and sprays and, most recently, Zyban have all been paraded as 'magic' cures. If any of them were effective, smoking would be about as rare today as that earlier form of nicotine addiction, snuff-taking. Given the number of disappointments most smokers have to endure in their quest to quit, it is not surprising they are resistant to pure marketing ploys. Easyway had become successful on its own merits as an effective quit-smoking method, not through clever marketing. A smoker will believe an endorsement given by another smoker. He won't believe someone who is being paid to tell him that such-and-such a product or approach works.

Nothing could be a substitute for a session with a trained Easyway therapist. Products, like books and videos, offered the promise of extending our reach towards smokers, but it was very difficult to ascertain how much they helped people to quit. I suspected that the people who had succeeded in stopping because of them were in a minority.

Initially the video had fulfilled my expectations, but it is easy to be impressed when you are ignorant of alternative approaches. Someone had given me a copy of a quit-smoking video fronted by actor Larry Hagman. At this time I was so tired that I would usually fall asleep after five minutes in front of the television, even when a programme was about something that interested me. The content of the verbal message in that quit smoking video was rubbish, but the methods used to convey it opened my eyes to what might be achieved with minimal dialogue and stunning images. Our video was dull and amateurish by comparison. Consisting of 90 percent me, preaching to the camera, it should have been sold as a sure cure for insomnia. The message was great, of course, but it was lost, the presentation such that people would not stay alert long enough to absorb it. I reached the unhappy conclusion that our video was a second-rate product. No amount of marketing would change this basic fact.

You might remember a TV advert about Remington razors in which Victor Kiam proclaims: 'I liked the product so much, I bought the company.' At the start of our collaboration Richard had made the same boast about Easyway. As it slowly dawned on him that it would take more than heavy advertising to turn the video into a money-spinner, he became noticeably less enthusiastic about it and Easyway in general. He seemed to lose interest, too, in our progress building up business at the new clinic in Birmingham, which Joyce and I were financing out of our own resources.

As the bad news piled up for Richard, so the tension increased at our regular board meetings. The first intimation we had that Richard was looking to cut his losses came at one of those meetings, when he announced that he no longer wanted such a prominent role in Easyway. His reason was that his father and Matt's had financial interests in tobacco companies and might be discomfited if it became known in City circles that their sons were involved in a campaign against nicotine addiction.

I had not met Messrs Kalms and Jacomb Snr, but I found it hard to believe that either gentleman would be embarrassed by such a revelation or be minded to pressurize his son. I was no tycoon, but could imagine that most successful businessmen would prefer their offspring to show initiative and be independently minded.

I could not understand Richard's change of attitude. For several months he had seemingly delighted in his role as front man, and had not so much as hinted at a potential conflict of interests. Now he wanted me to take over the marketing side. I refused point blank. As someone with no expertise in marketing and even less faith in its benefits, I was hardly the right person. I had made no secret of my priorities or my opinion of the video. The way forward was to concentrate on what worked for the majority of smokers: face-to-face sessions conducted by trained therapists. Instead of wasting money advertising the video, we should concentrate our efforts on developing the work Joyce and I had embarked on and build a network of clinics.

I thought my argument had struck home when, at the next board meeting, Richard proposed that we sell franchises. The price tag would be £5,000 per franchise, which would include me spending three months training each franchisee. I had no problem with the principle of selling franchises, only with how it was done. There had to be safeguards. It had taken over a year to train Roy. Admittedly, he had been a slow learner, but even Robin had required six months of my time. Nobody could become a competent Easyway therapist in just three months, and to pretend otherwise would have been tantamount to perpetrating a fraud on the franchisees and their clients. There was also the matter of ensuring the area covered by the franchise was large enough to support the franchisee. Having sweat blood and tears to build up the reputation of Easyway, Joyce and I did not want to see it become discredited. I insisted on having the final say on whether a franchisee had reached the level of competence necessary for the proper practice of the method.

Richard was furious. Both of us were in a bind. Even as managing director and the major shareholder in the company, he could not sell franchises without my cooperation. Equally, I could not open new clinics without Richard's permission because of the company's ownership of the intellectual rights to Easyway. This stand off lasted several months, during which time our relationship deteriorated to the stage where Richard would not talk to me, and all communication between us had to be conducted through Matt.

I suppose it is inevitable in such situations that you start counting men. It was a fair bet that Matt and Piers would side with Richard. That left Robin. I decided to confide in him. I told him of my misgivings about the direction Richard was mapping out, and outlined the problems we were having. Apart from wanting to gauge his reaction, it seemed only fair to warn him that his spell at Easyway might come to an abrupt end. Robin had reached the point in his training where he was sitting in on my sessions in Birmingham, and so we were regularly driving up together. The journey was of long enough duration for us to progress beyond the usual niceties to exchange ideas on a range of subjects. Our conversations convinced me that his motivation and mind-set were fully aligned with my own. I was certain of where his loyalties lay when he told me that the debt of gratitude he felt towards me personally for helping him to stop smoking meant that he could not support any party about whom I had serious doubts.

When I had this conversation with Robin I had little idea my dispute with Richard would escalate as it did. In an attempt to bring it to an amicable conclusion, I offered to take over the company and to recoup all Richard's losses out of future profits. He responded by instructing his solicitors to sue me on the grounds that I was not acting in the best interests of the company. The only fortuitous aspect of this writ was its timing. Robin had reached the end of his training and was already running Birmingham. He ended up taking over a good deal more as the dispute escalated and demanded all my energies.

I like to think that I weigh situations by applying logic to them. What did my logic tell me about the latest turn of events? Simply, that Richard had a case. After all, companies are meant to make profits. The franchises he proposed would have recouped his losses in the short term. My logic also told me that we would be up against top lawyers, because Richard could afford the best. I was well aware of the dictum that when it comes to court cases the winner is not the man with the best argument but with the best lawyers.

I cannot recall a more stressful period of my life. It seemed that whatever course of action I took, one way or another Joyce and I would be plunged into the depths of bankruptcy, financial or moral. If I gave into Richard's pressure, and let him market and sell franchises as he saw fit, I would be saved financial ruin but at the cost of turning Easyway into a travesty of itself. If I fought the case and lost, Easyway would still be doomed and I would be penniless; as the case would be heard in the High Court, I could expect to be landed with costs approaching £100,000 for each day of the hearing.

The decision I arrived at was not mine alone. Joyce and I were a partnership and her opinion counted. But she knew I would follow my conscience, trust in British justice and fight my corner. She agreed that penury would be preferable to selling out my principles and all we had worked for together.

Fortunately, we did not have to put our resolution to the test, because Richard eventually agreed to settle out of court. I shall be forever grateful to him for that. Under the terms of the settlement, I bought out Piers, Matt and Richard, thus gaining control over the company and, absolutely crucially from my perspective, regaining complete control of the intellectual rights to Easyway. In effect, Richard walked away, leaving us with a very expensive lease in Hanover Square for premises we did not need, and a company whose accounts and sales admin were in chaos. Robin, Joyce and I pooled our expertise to sort out the muddle.

The most positive aspect of the Kalms episode was that it forced me to examine my position and to ask hard questions of myself. Easyway was almost a decade old and as fresh as the day I had formulated it. I was nearing sixty, and in a handful of years would have to make way for someone younger. Why wait? The future of the company was already taking shape under Robin's stewardship and I liked what I saw. Joyce and I agreed to confirm Robin in the role he was already filling, as Managing Director of Easyway (International) Ltd. It came as a huge relief to formally put Easyway in the hands of a man dedicated to spreading its word and, more importantly, upholding the principles on which it was established. The future of Easyway was secure.

Reaching the Parts Others Can't

The success of Easyway has led some people to believe that I am some sort of general healer or miracle worker. I am sure that the principles of Easyway have wider applications than just smoking, and when given the opportunity I have tried to prove this. Some requests were unusual: a professional golfer who could take the club back but not bring it down again; a young woman who had a compunction to pull hairs out of her head. I agreed to treat both. A lord enquired if I could cure his wife of snoring. I declined that particular challenge, but in cases where I thought I might be able to help, I would agree to see the person. As much of this work was experimental, I refused a fee and warned that a cure was not guaranteed.

Usually the problem I was asked to solve was one of substance addiction, typically alcohol or heroin. Invariably the people who approached me had failed with the usual treatments. My success in helping them made me realize that Easyway is effective for all sorts of drug addiction. Alcohol addiction, in particular, figured prominently as a topic in the letters I was receiving, with many correspondents urging me to write a book about it. I saw no point in allowing myself to become distracted by another addiction until I had succeeded in persuading the opinion formers and law makers that Easyway is the most effective method for curing smokers.

In my most recent book *The Onlyway*, I had included chapters on both drug and alcohol addiction, and that was about as far as I was prepared to go for the moment. Researching and writing that book had taken two years and left me not wanting to write again for a very long time, if ever.

Then, seemingly out of the blue, one of our most dynamic therapists asked my permission to use the Easyway method to write a book on alcohol. He declared that he had been an alcoholic and that his real ambition in life was to cure the world of alcoholism. This seemed an ideal solution: someone who was an ex-alcoholic who understood the method. I agreed to him using the Easyway principles on condition that I vetted the script before it was published. As far as I was concerned, this would be an Easyway book.

A year later the manuscript arrived. I was horrified by what I read. Quite apart from the frequent use of unnecessarily foul language, the structure was badly flawed. After a great deal of discussion, I agreed to let him try again. Another year passed. What I then received was not a revised manuscript but a finished book, entitled *The Easy Way to Stop Drinking*, with its author taking the entire credit for the ideas contained therein. His 'original' ideas were blatant copies of the principles of Easyway. With the book was enclosed a letter, requesting my endorsement. I might have agreed if on closer scrutiny I had not discovered that the published book was as badly flawed as the draft I had rejected.

In the two years since agreeing to him writing the book, I had told my publisher and interested members of the public that an Easyway title about alcohol was being produced. To make good my promise, I had now to sit down and write the book myself.

I had come across many alcoholics in my smoking clinics apart from in those one-to-one ad hoc sessions. Many in this latter group were fully paid up members of the awkward squad: angry, aggressive and difficult to communicate with. I regarded these people as ex-alcoholics, because they had been through AA and as far as I was aware no longer had a problem with alcohol. They saw their situation very differently, and this vision distorted their approach to Easyway. I remember one lady in particular who said to me:

'I've been a smoker for over 30 years. How dare you suggest that I can be free of it after just four hours!'

I couldn't understand her attitude. I had been recommended to her by several of her friends, all of them long-term heavy smokers who had left the clinic after the first session as happy non-smokers. If they could do it, why couldn't she? Not surprisingly, given her frame of mind, she did not succeed after one session and had to come back for a second. It transpired that she was an ex-alcoholic, and in her mind still an alcoholic. She regularly attended Alcoholics Anonymous meetings and was ingrained with the notion that there is no cure for alcoholism, let alone an immediate and easy one.

I did not think it fair to rely solely on the impressions of alcoholics I had formed at my clinics, and decided to attend AA meetings. The experience was an eye-opener. I was expecting to find people there who were living at the margins of society, whereas the vast majority of attendees came across as educated, intelligent, articulate people. Some had been managers or successful business people before falling into the alcohol trap. Many others had become successful again after dragging themselves away from dependency. In some cases members hadn't touched a drop of alcohol for many years, and yet they were still turning up at meetings.

Regardless of where in the country I went, the pattern of each AA meeting seemed to be the same. One member would give an opening address in which he (or she) described his decline into the pit and emphasized the continuing help he received from AA in his recovery. After the opening address the other attendees would stand up one by one and tell their stories. Each speaker would be listened to in silence, almost with reverence. I cannot remember a single interruption. Some of these stories were truly heart-rending, personal tragedies on an epic scale. In such confessional situations there is always a danger of truth being sacrificed in the interests of a good show, and I sensed this in several accounts. On occasions I was reminded of the Monty Python sketch in which several overweight, dinner-jacketed businessmen, clutching brandies and Havanas, compete over the humbleness of their beginnings:

'You lived in a coal shed? You were lucky! Us eight kids were brought up in a shoe-box!'
'Did your shoe-box have a lid?'
'Aye!'
'You were lucky. Our lid was stolen!'

Without exception, each speaker would commence his story with the words:

'I am an alcoholic.'

He or she might just as well said, 'I'm just one drink away from alcoholism.' This thinking struck me as being very negative and certainly the atmosphere at these meetings was generally morbid. It must be difficult to enjoy life if, sooner or later, you are expecting to be back at some terrible square one. The 'recovering' alcoholics who had abstained for years seemed almost as miserable as the people who were still trying to haul themselves out of the pit. Some of these people had not touched a drop of alcohol in 20 years, and yet to look at them you would have thought they were still in its thrall.

Another cause of disquiet was the language used. Although unfailingly courteous to one another, they spat bile and venom when mentioning people called 'normal' drinkers. Perhaps being part of a group brings out the worst in us in this respect. My stint in the RAF dramatically reduced my vocabulary, with even short sentences containing more expletives than proper words. I came to the conclusion that, almost without exception, the people I met at these AA meetings were miserable, angry with themselves and life, even the ones who no longer drank.

Although I was impressed by much of what I witnessed, I could not avoid the conclusion that AA, for all the good it has done in saving lives from ruination, does not fully understand the alcohol trap. Like most diseases, alcoholism is progressive. People do not suddenly become heavy drinkers, any more than they suddenly become heavy smokers. They work up to it from a seemingly benign start. Fortunately, most people who drink do not become chronic alcoholics. This situation creates the illusion that those people who do become chronic alcoholics have some inherent flaw in their character that marks them out from 'normal' drinkers. Why else do so-called 'recovering' alcoholics express such resentment of 'normal' drinkers if it is not because they are envious of their position and want to return to this perceived state of grace? All addictions tend to render their victims incapable of admitting they have a problem. For most of their drinking lives people with an alcohol problem will deny they are other than 'normal' drinkers. When they finally face up to it, they cast themselves in a totally different mould. In reality those envied 'normal' drinkers are in denial about their own situation of being in the early stages of the same disease.

The alcoholic is right to see alcoholism as a disease, but wrong to believe he is incapable of cure. And by 'cure' I mean someone who is free of the need or desire to consume alcohol. That person may not necessarily be cured immediately of the physical effects of alcoholism, but they are completely cured of the disease itself. You might well argue that no one can ever know they are permanently cured, hence the fear of those AA members. They can if they understand how the confidence trick works, and the illusions on which it is based.

Alcohol is more complicated than nicotine because its benefits are based on a double illusion. The first is that alcohol quenches your thirst. In fact, it does the complete opposite and actually dehydrates you. Why else does it rarely take more than one glass of water, even on a hot day, to quench your thirst, whereas you can drink alcohol all evening in winter and still feel thirsty? You will also probably wake up in the middle of the night with a throat resembling a dried-up river-bed.

The other effect of alcohol is that it inebriates you. Inebriation is thought of as a kind of analgesic for the mind. If you have a problem, you can drown your sorrows by becoming inebriated. No one is stupid enough to believe that inebriation actually helps to solve problems, any more than an ostrich actually buries its head in sand to make itself invisible to a perceived threat.

And yet the majority of drinkers still consume alcohol in the belief that it will. Can you think of a single instance of alcohol solving a problem, either yours or anyone else's? I've no doubt that you know of social occasions that have been ruined because someone drank too much. Alcohol has the effect of altering every sense we rely on for survival.

So why is it that we can see the ostrich analogy so clearly, yet most of us continue to delude ourselves that we get some pleasure or crutch from alcohol? Why, several years after conducting successful experimental sessions with alcoholics, did I continue to drink and why was my intake increasing? Was it because I didn't truly believe there was no genuine pleasure to be had from drinking alcohol? Not so. Just as with nicotine, I knew I had no need for it until I started consuming it. I could remember clearly the foul taste of those first few pints, and thinking: 'Do adults really like drinking this muck? I'd much rather stick to lemonade!'

But only children drink lemonade. Adults drink alcohol. And so the brainwashing started to seep into my consciousness. I was influenced by it from an early age, as are most of us. We are being prepared for the trap. Who can visualize a wedding or a party without alcohol? When someone has a nasty shock or is chilled, brandy is administered. The inexperienced can be weaned onto the 'pleasure' of the majority by having their alcoholic drink sweetened with sugar or mixed with lemonade. Given the influence we are subjected to it is surprising that a small percentage of people do actually avoid falling into the trap, probably because they've been brought up with or by someone who had a serious alcohol problem.

It is very difficult to convince drinkers that enjoying the taste of alcohol is not the reason why they drink. Pure alcohol tastes awful and is lethal, which is why we dilute it with water, mixers and sweeteners. It's even more difficult to convince drinkers that the inebriated state does not equal happiness. As well as being a powerful poison, alcohol is also a depressant. The reason we think it makes us happy is because most of our heavy drinking is done in leisure time, on happy occasions with our friends. Smokers get no particular pleasure from smoking when they are allowed to smoke and take it for granted. It is only when they try to quit, or are prevented from smoking, that they feel miserable and deprived. The obvious conclusion to draw from this is that smoking must provide a great crutch or pleasure. This is wrong. The same error is made with alcohol. If you consciously drink alcohol and try to analyse the pleasure, you will fail. However, if you believe that social occasions cannot be enjoyed without drinking, you will be miserable without a drink in your hand.

Drinking differs from smoking in two important respects. Smoking is a completely unnatural pastime. No matter how much we are brainwashed, we instinctively know that it is both unnatural and unhealthy. Drinking is not only perfectly natural but essential. We can survive longer without food than we can without water. There are few greater pleasures than slaking a thirst on a hot day after strenuous physical activity. The pleasure is almost as great if you quench that thirst with a glass of beer as a glass of water. We need to be aware that the water content of that glass of beer is probably ten to twenty times greater than its alcohol content. It is the water content that quenches your thirst not the alcohol. Would even the heaviest drinker attempt to quench his thirst with a pint of whisky?

Since the connection between nicotine and lung cancer was established, smoking has gone from being a highly sociable habit to a decidedly anti-social one. The mystery nowadays is to imagine how it could ever have been regarded otherwise; a pipe-smoker in a crowded lift is about as welcome as a fart in a space suit. However, drinking is still regarded as both normal and sociable, as long as it is not combined with driving. It is difficult to believe that not many years ago a host would have been regarded as remiss if he did not persuade a guest to have just one more for the road.

This is the real problem with drinking. It is still very much a part of our culture. Just as men who didn't smoke were once viewed with suspicion, so, today, non-drinkers can be made to feel uncomfortable when they are in the company of drinkers. It takes just one non-drinker behaving normally among a group of people who are behaving stupidly under the influence of alcohol to attract accusations of party-pooperism. If you have ever been the only sober person in the presence of a giggling group of drunks, you will know that it is impossible to enjoy yourself. The worst part isn't the foul language, the insincere flattery and overt emotions or even the slurred, repetitive gobbledegook, but the sheer boredom of trying to make conversation with brains that are smashed.

I continued to drink long after I had reached the conclusion that, like smoking, alcohol is just another of Western society's confidence tricks. I had no reason to deny myself. Whereas smokers instinctively know throughout their lives that smoking is both stupid and unnatural, drinking seems entirely natural. While a drinker is at the stage of the fly that has just started to enjoy the nectar it has found in the pitcher plant, it doesn't matter that the pleasure or crutch he derives from alcohol is illusory.

Alcohol was causing me no particular problems, mentally, physically or financially. True, very occasionally I would become one of those giggling, mindless bores, and sometimes I would ask Joyce to drive because I had had too much. Many things in life that we do knowingly are not really good for us. When we binge on that Christmas dinner we know what we are doing isn't particularly healthy, that we'll probably need some indigestion tablets and that we won't be able to move out of that armchair for the next three hours. But, hey, what's the harm now and again?

My descent into chain-smoking was a very rapid affair and no way could I kid myself that I hadn't got a problem with cigarettes. However, my slide down the pitcher plant of alcohol was slow, prolonged and easy to deny. Even when I was deep down in the pitcher plant and knew there was only one direction to go, I denied that I had a drink problem. In a sense I hadn't – a problem ceases to be a problem if you don't let it worry you!

My drinking career started with shandys at dances and weddings. I quickly progressed to brown ales, then discovered that 'real' men drank draught beer. I embarrassed my father by ordering half a pint of brown ale at his local. He insisted I drink a pint of mild ale. It took me until closing time to finish it.

My education took another giant stride forward on the

day I was allowed to buy my first round. The occasion was the local's annual day trip to Brighton when we stopped at a famous half-way house called The Chinese Gardens. I struggled across with a tray full of pints of mild to where my dad and his friends were waiting expectantly. Their censure could not have been more severe if I had been about to hand round pints of poison.

The pints were in jars (a glass with a handle), tantamount to plastic cups in the eyes of my dad and his friends, whose custom it was to drink out of clear, straight glasses.

Just as with tobacco, no matter how foul alcohol tastes initially, if you persist with a particular type you will learn to enjoy it, or, more accurately, to cope with it. I was drinking pints of mild for about two years before National Service. I always regarded it as a rather insipid drink. I cannot remember actually enjoying it, that is until I stopped drinking it. In the Midlands, where I did my basic RAF training, the local mild was a Burton brew, reputed to be the best beer in the country. I couldn't wait to get back to Putney for a decent pint of Young's. When I did finally get home, I went straight round to the pub, still in uniform, and waited for it to open. The publican immediately recognized me as Johnny Carr's son and insisted on buying me a pint. I was salivating with expectation as I watched him slowly pull the pint. I took a deep quaff. It tasted awful.

'Cheap bastard,' I thought, 'he's only bought it because he knows it's off.'

I said: 'There's something wrong with this!' He denied it. I asked him to sample it. After swallowing far more than he needed to, he concluded that it was a perfectly good pint.

I would not take his word. As each new customer came in, I got him to taste the suspect beer. Not one of them had the guts to confirm there was something wrong with it. I was so pleased when my father finally arrived. I knew I could rely on him to be honest, even if his verdict upset the publican. I couldn't wait to be vindicated. My father downed what was now left of the pint, confirmed there was nothing wrong with it and immediately ordered another round.

Having spent eight weeks pining for a pint of Young's, I had drunk one and was now pining for a pint of Burton's. My taste had changed. I learned an important lesson that night: there is no such thing as good or bad tasting alcoholic drinks. Like your mother's cooking, whatever you are brought up on tastes the best.

When I was working at Peat Marwick after National Service, I got into the habit of joining several other employees for lunch in a nearby pub. These were middle to upper class people. Middle-class beer drinkers drink bitter, not mild. Ask them why they prefer bitter and they'll tell you that it tastes better.

My dictionary defines bitter as:

'Tasting sharp like quinine or aspirin, not sweet.'

This is not very helpful. It assumes that most of us have lived in mosquito-infested environs, have caught malaria and know what quinine tastes like. I have yet to meet anyone who has tasted quinine. Practically all of us have tasted aspirin at some time in our lives. A better description of bitter would be, 'like sucking a lemon'.

Whichever definition you choose, bitter is definitely a taste to avoid. There are literally millions of people who drink bitter in the belief that they do so because it tastes nice. I have yet to meet a single person who takes aspirin because it tastes nice.

I pride myself on learning by my mistakes. When I bought my first round of pints of bitter one lunch break, I insisted to the barman that he use straight, clear glasses and not the jars he was reaching for. No way was I falling for that one again. When I handed round the pints, I was met with the same looks of horror from the bitter drinkers as I had received from the mild drinkers. Bitter drinkers like their tipple in a jar. How pernickety can you get? But in no time at all, I could only drink mild from a straight clear glass and bitter from a pint jug.

On special occasions, when they were feeling particularly flush, my dad and his friends would drink mild and bitter. I have never drunk a pint of mild and bitter in my life. Because I don't like mixing drinks? No, because I wouldn't know whether to drink it out of a straight glass or a jug!

The single pint of bitter during lunch soon increased to two or three but without them having any obvious adverse effects. During the six months I spent in the general office at Peat Marwick the manager was a man named Marshall, who would arrive late every morning, bleary-eyed and reeking of stale beer. He would mumble to himself until lunch time then go out for three hours and come back in an even worse state. It must have been blatantly obvious to all twenty partners of the firm that Mr Marshall contributed nothing but confusion. I could not understand why they kept him on and in hindsight the reason can only have been because of the years of loyal service he had given in the past.

Anyone who has been unfortunate enough to suffer from chronic alcoholism will know that it is not possible to exaggerate the depths to which you can sink. Did I ever picture myself becoming like Mr Marshall? It never entered my head. Sure there were times when I got hopelessly drunk in the early days, but each time the experience was so horrible it would keep me sober for months. Apart from Christmas parties, I cannot remember being incapable of doing my work. Mind you, it depends what you mean by incapable. When I reached the stage of having several drinks to make up my liquid lunch I would ensure my workload in the afternoons did not require above-average levels of concentration.

Several companies I worked for provided very good free canteen lunches for staff, and I took advantage of this perk. Not drinking alcohol at lunchtimes did not leave me feeling deprived. For a period, my drinking was confined to after work with colleagues. I still had no feeling of deriving genuine pleasure from alcohol. Its main attraction was the distraction and company it provided. At weekends, I could partake of my real pleasure, golf.

In my early golfing days, after the game, I would go straight home to the Sunday roast, until one day:

'Aren't you going to buy me a drink? Come on, don't be unsociable. After all, you've won my money!'

I could barely afford to play golf let alone treat the old fogey who chided me with this remark. But how could a new member ignore such a hint, especially as this particular old fogey was the club captain? Of course he would be embarrassed if I didn't allow him to reciprocate.

I can't remember making a conscious decision to stay for a drink after every match but it soon became the norm for me to have two or three. Occasionally I would stay on for a frame or two of snooker as well. In the winter, before teeing off, I would join some of the other members for a brandy or two, just to get the blood circulating. Of course they were large ones, and naturally we continued the habit in the summer. If I was having a particularly bad round, I would look forward to another brandy, or two, at the half-way stage. For some reason the bad rounds multiplied out of all proportion to the good ones. I can't think why. I used to win quite a few competitions when I first joined the club.

Some of the lads used to carry flasks around with them. I promised myself that I would never have a flask: it was the first step to alcoholism. But my daughter gave me one on my birthday. It was beautiful, made of silver and had my initials engraved on it. I couldn't hurt her feelings by not using it. Actually it turned out to be very useful, a bit like my PC; I don't know how I used to manage without one. Lovely as it was, my flask was on the small side. Naturally it was polite to offer it around. Amazingly, some of the younger members didn't have a flask and those who did weren't so free with theirs as I was with mine. For some inexplicable reason mine always seemed to be the first to empty. I solved this problem by buying a larger one.

I used to despise the old fogeys when I first joined the golf club, and characterized them as rude, irritable, bad-tempered old men, with large red noses and bleary red eyes to match, who sat around sipping whisky and water.

The highlight of their year was if they could catch the steward topping up their glass with a Teacher's instead of a Bell's or vice versa. They would make so much fuss you would think he had topped them up with poison. Come to think of it, he had. I did not recognize my own gradual deterioration into old fogeydom.

My drinking pattern changed yet again with the demise of Lines Brothers and the start of my new life with Joyce. We were so busy building our business and later renovating houses that liquid lunches were out of the question. By the end of the day we were usually physically exhausted and content to stretch out and watch TV. On my rare trips to the golf club, I would play a round and happily return to Joyce rather than stay and drink with other golfers. Our main entertainment was a meal out with friends. At the time I would have described myself as one of those 'normal' drinkers who enjoys a glass of wine with his evening meal. In truth, my intake was more like a bottle than one glass. Joyce has rarely drunk more than one glass of wine, and even then she mixes it with lemonade. I am convinced the only reason she drinks alcohol at all is so as not to make other people feel uncomfortable.

Have you noticed how in old Hollywood films every apartment has a well stocked bar? I suppose it's one of those clichés for good living, a sign of chic, that sticks in our psyche. In several of the houses we renovated we were faced with troublesome spaces that were too small to do anything with other than convert them into a bar. The house in Raynes Park had one such nook, which we duly converted into a very attractive mahogany topped bar. As this was to be our home as well as the first Easyway clinic, friends gave us house-warming presents, including automatic drinks dispensers and cut glasses. Just as you stock a refrigerator with food, so you stock a bar with booze, and I made sure ours was very well stocked. We weren't in the position of our parents who could only afford drinks in the house at Christmas.

Ironically, the success of Easyway sent me sliding down into the alcohol pit again. After talking to smokers for a solid ten hours, I would give a sigh of relief as the last one left and within minutes be pouring myself a whisky-mac.

At one time if you had put an open box of chocolates in front of me I would have scoffed the lot, whereas if they were out of sight they were also out of mind. I was a bit like that with alcohol. Where was the harm in just one drink, I told myself? I should have known I would be like a kid in a sweet shop, incapable of not indulging. The drink was there and available. I was caught in the typical drug addict's conflict:

'I've worked hard all day. I've earned a reward. I would like a drink. Just one, you understand.'

'But you know alcohol isn't good for you.'

'I know, but surely there's no harm in just one drink?'

'Of course there isn't. But you never do have just one drink.'

Alcohol makes you thirsty. You read the sign and tell yourself you want another drink. The sensible half of your brain should kick in and say:

'I told you one wouldn't be enough!'

But that first drink has also partially inebriated you, lessening your awareness of the consequences and lowering your resistance. Dean Martin summed up the drinker's situation brilliantly:

'I need one drink. Just one and it will make a new man of me. Then the new man, he needs a drink.'

Such is the nature of the beast. In no time at all, I was drinking the whole evening. I had no problems, no stress. Life was all honey and roses. Although I fully understood the nature of the alcohol trap, I did not perceive my position in it as a problem. I could fly away whenever I wanted to! Such is the power of denial.

One of the cornerstones of Easyway is the danger of substitutes, such as food, chewing gum, drink or NRT. Just as you don't need to search for another disease to replace a bout of flu, substitutes merely support the illusion that you are making a sacrifice and then the substitute itself becomes a problem. Was my drinking a form of substitution for nicotine? No way. When I was a smoker I had to smoke all day. If I was substituting, I would have had to drink all day!

I had no problem with drink, but Joyce was convinced that I had. Whenever the subject of drink came up, she would say:

'You tell me there are no advantages to drinking alcohol. If you truly believe that, why do you drink all night, every night?'

I would reply: 'Do you believe there are no genuine advantages to drinking alcohol?'

She would always agree that there aren't. I would then ask her why she drank alcohol. Her answer was always:

'To be sociable!'

Such is the power of denial. Joyce always pointed out that I drank much more than she did. Isn't that just another ingenious aspect of drug addiction? We all know someone who is deeper in the pit than we are, and convince ourselves that we would quit before we reached their stage of addiction.

The truth is that no one ever makes a conscious decision to become a smoker for life, or an alcoholic, or a heroin addict or any other form of drug addict. None of us needs these drugs until we fall into the trap. The nature of all drug addiction is to keep us in the trap once we have fallen into it. I was aware that alcohol provided no advantages whatsoever, but equally I believed it was not a problem. Not until I started researching *The Easy Way to Control Alcohol*, and came to the conclusion that it was indeed a problem, did the scales fall from my eyes, enabling me to look at myself honestly.

Going Global

In the early days at Raynes Park I soon discovered that nationality had a bearing on whether or not a smoker would be successful with Easyway. Smokers from countries in northern latitudes were generally more successful than those from southern climes. The success rate was high among the Scandinavians, Germans and Dutch, whereas the French, Italians and Spanish did markedly less well. We speculated on possible reasons for this disparity, and reached the conclusion that the attitude to smoking is far more tolerant in the south than the north and that this affects the ability of clients to quit. In addition, clients from northerly countries generally had a better grasp of English.

When we compared the success rates of native English speakers against those who were not, we found a further difference. Even foreign clients with excellent English would tend to concentrate on the literal meaning of words while failing to understand their true significance. It can be so easy to miss the point in another language, especially one as complex as English, which abounds in ambiguities and relies on the individual's facility for picking up on subtle nuances of meaning. It is hardly surprising some of our foreign clients struggled. I gave them as much help as I could while recognizing that I could not entirely make up for their linguistic shortcomings. Many of these clients had travelled thousands of miles just to attend a session, and I felt very bad when they went away obviously still wrestling with the concept of Easyway. With some of them it must have seemed as though their last chance of escape had gone.

It has always been a key objective to bring Easyway to every smoker, wherever they are. And by Easyway I mean the method as I conceived and developed it, not some watered down or otherwise adulterated version. When Easyway was still in its infancy we were receiving letters from former clients expressing interest in becoming therapists. Very soon we were also receiving letters from overseas clients wanting to set up clinics in their own countries. The first of these requests we took seriously came from a young Dutch woman called Eveline de Mooij, who wanted to start a clinic in Holland. I was rather dubious about the prospects of Easyway in other countries, except where English is the first language. However, her success at the clinic, and subsequently in translating my first book so well that it became the No 1 bestseller in Holland, made me realize that Easyway is a universal method. The only proviso is that the people who present it fully understand its principles and are capable of expressing them accurately in their own language.

Where Eveline first dared to tread others soon followed, so that by 2003 we had clinics in 19 countries outside the UK. In cultures where smoking has been so accepted as to be considered the norm, I have had serious reservations about Easyway's chances of success, and certainly the therapists in these places have faced a greater challenge than where society is disapproving of smokers.

However, even where the omens are unpromising, such as in Spain, Italy, Portugal, Ecuador and Colombia, Easyway is making inroads into smoker numbers.

Any lingering conceit I might have retained about my importance to the ongoing development of Easyway has been eroded by its success as it continues to grow. The principal reason for this is the commitment of the people who are taking it forward. Easyway has never been purely a commodity or service to be bought and sold, and to be effective it has to be presented by people who believe wholeheartedly in it as well as fully understand its principles. This is rare in a world where how much you sell is more important than what you sell. Because they share common values and aims the therapists who make up the Easyway organization are a close-knit bunch, despite the physical distance separating them. Since the advent of email this has been no barrier to communication and the sharing of information. We now have a full-time head of business development who liaises between clinics and monitors their performance to ensure that Easyway continues to live up to its name.

It has been suggested to me that the expansion of Easyway must have been greatly assisted by the fact that many high-profile people have sought my help. A number of them have indeed attended my sessions. If I look at a roll call, I am deeply impressed: Marti Caine, Patrick Cargill, Johnny Cash, Christopher Cazenove, Julie Christie, Fish, Frederick Forsyth, Emma Freud, Leslie Grantham, Robin Jackman, Mathew Kelly, Mark Knopfler, Rula Lenska, Ian Maxwell, John Cougar Mellencamp, Jenni Murray, John Sessions, Nina Simone, Dennis Waterman, Ruby Wax and Susannah York, to name but a few.

All of them came of their own accord or as a result of a recommendation. The sessions I had with them were in the main quite unremarkable: we would sit and chat for four hours and afterwards I would never see them or hear from them again, other than through thank-you letters, television or the radio.

One of the biggest surprises I received from a celebrity had absolutely nothing to do with quitting smoking. Several times during our session together Rula Lenska commented that I reminded her of someone but that she couldn't put her finger on who it was. Eventually she did, and shouted excitedly: 'I've got it!' I braced myself for the inevitable 'Matt Monroe' comparison and was completely nonplussed when out came, 'Charlton Heston!' Rula's companion, fellow actor Dennis Waterman, roared with laughter. By no stretch of the imagination have I ever looked like Charlton Heston, even if she was making the comparison to his contemporary self, 30 long years on from his Ben Hur days. It stands as the most flattering compliment I have received.

Incidentally, meeting Dennis took me back to my days at Wandsworth Grammar where I had the misfortune of coming up against his brother, Peter, in the boxing ring. A few years after pulverizing me he became British and European champion at welterweight.

I was always nervous when a celebrity was due, especially in the early days when I suspected that inside every 'name' there was some prima donna fighting to get out. Gradually the suspicion was replaced by self-imposed pressure. I knew that if I could help a celebrity to quit our combined success would speed the spreading of the word about Easyway. When Ruby Wax made an appointment I had several sleepless nights beforehand. Although a fan of hers for years, I was terrified that I wouldn't be able to help her if she didn't allow me to get a word in. I need not have worried. She turned out to be the ideal client. She looked relaxed, made me feel relaxed and absorbed everything I said, only occasionally putting a pertinent question when I failed to make myself clear. Over the years she has been a great advocate of our cause, for which I am exceedingly grateful.

The vast majority of the celebrities I have helped came across as intelligent, sensitive people, and in some instances quite unlike the image they projected on stage or screen. When Johnny Cash, a singer I had long admired, asked me to go up to Sheffield, where he was giving a concert, to help him, I was honoured, delighted and not a little star-struck. The man was a legend. The delight dissipated as he ushered me into his hotel suite. He looked and sounded terrible. It was difficult to believe he was able to perform in such a debilitated state.

I asked the question I put to all my clients:

'What prompted you to quit now?'

He said: 'I know it's been killing me for years. But I made the decision after one of my shows recently. A group of us were having a drink and a chat and I ran out of cigarettes. Other people were offering them to me, but I felt naked without my own. I offered to buy a pack from one of the others but it was his last and he wouldn't sell it to me. I offered him a hundred dollars for it. It wasn't that I was trying to be flash but I needed those cigarettes. He said, "I don't want your hundred dollars. If you need them that bad, you can have 'em." Everyone was staring at me as if I was mad. It made me realize the grip cigarettes held over me.'

Johnny recommended me to several of his friends who

flew over from the States and from various other parts of the world to attend the clinic. One of them, musician John Cougar Mellencamp, was forced to change his plans at the last minute and could not get to London. Instead he arranged for Joyce and I to fly by Concorde to New York where we met up.

In June 2001, on being asked for his reaction to the news of George Harrison's death from cancer, John Mellencamp said:

'This smoking is bullshit, isn't it? I hate it. I'd like to quit tonight, but, you know, I'm weak. What do you want me to say?'

Failure always hurts. But some failures hurt more than others.

One morning Joyce interrupted a group session and asked me to leave the therapy room. This was unprecedented. Once a session was underway it progressed without interruption to its conclusion. She was clearly in a state of excitement. I wondered what momentous event could have occurred.

She said: 'Kerry Packer's secretary is on the phone. He is offering to pay you ten thousand pounds if you can stop him smoking for a month!'

Even today that is a great deal of money. Fifteen years ago it seemed a lot more.

I said: 'Terrific! So what's the problem?'

The problem was that the Australian media mogul did not want to come to the clinic. He wanted me to treat him in his suite at the Savoy. What's more he wanted me to do so immediately. There followed one of those ridiculous situations I had unwittingly been involved in regularly when I worked at Tri-ang. You ask your secretary to get Mr X on the line. Mr X's secretary says,

'Who wants him?' and on being told follows up with, 'OK, put Mr Carr on.' My secretary says, 'I can't do that. You need to put Mr X on first.' There then follows a contest between the two secretaries as to whose boss is the more powerful. This is very important to them because their own status depends on the result. Meanwhile, as both Mr X and I are hanging on waiting to be connected, we are wondering why the telephone system is so congested. It took me years to discover the reason.

Anyway, back to Kerry Packer. I was very surprised to receive this call and also pleased. A few years earlier, in 1989, he had tried to take over British American Tobacco with a view to fully exploiting the potential of the business in the third world. His bid failed, thankfully. In regions of the world already blighted by numerous ills, natural and man-made, a push for further growth by one of the big tobacco companies is not the kind of development that will help the situation of the indigenous people in the long run. I took it as a good sign that Packer, reputedly a heavy smoker, now wanted to address his personal problem with smoking.

I asked Joyce to 'phone his secretary and explain that I was in the middle of a session, that I had another group session after it and that I would contact him as soon as I was free. I said too that he would be far more likely to succeed if he came to the clinic.

The secretary came back with: 'Mr Packer wants to know how much these other people are paying you?'

Up to this point I had been an admirer of Kerry Packer. As a cricket lover I had supported his move to break the grip of the vested interests that had controlled and stifled the game for decades. But I took exception to the assumption that money can buy everything and everybody. I asked Joyce to tell him that he should pretend he's the Christmas turkey and get stuffed.

Joyce remonstrated with me: 'Allen, for once in your life swallow your pride. We'd be mad to throw away the chance of making £10,000!'

I complied and let her arrange a compromise with the secretary. At 5 o'clock that evening, having already spent eight hours working, I made my way to the Savoy. In case you are thinking that the prospect of £10,000 had sweetened my temper, you would be wrong. Several factors had already convinced me that I would not be able to help Kerry Packer quit for a day let alone a month.

First, to give the therapy away from the clinic is equivalent to asking a surgeon to remove someone's appendix in the local pub rather than in an operating theatre. Second, he would not be getting the full session. He had only time for a shortened version of the therapy and I had no idea how effective that would be. Third, I am literally drained after two full sessions in a day and could not possibly be at my best, especially on a hot summer's day, which this was. These negatives had been explained to Mr Packer, but he had refused to consider them as important or indeed relevant. If this was indicative of his open mindedness, it did not bode well. I set out for our 'session' feeling physically and mentally down, unhappy with the situation and with myself for agreeing to pander to what seemed like a rich man's whim.

When I got to the hotel I was sent up to his suite where I was received by an exceedingly attractive young woman, her long legs shown off to advantage by a skimpy mini-skirt. I was allowed to get just inside the door and then was told to wait. I could see the big man stretched out on a settee, his attention divided between giving instructions to two other secretaries and watching a game of tennis live from Wimbledon. An acknowledgement of my presence would have been gratifying, even more so an offer of some refreshment after the exertions of my journey. I was a sorry sight and perspiring as freely as the two players slugging it out on the television screen.

In the corner of the room I spied an assortment of drinks on a table and asked no one in particular if I could help myself to a glass of water. I took a dismissive wave of the hand from the settee as assent. While I drank my water, he continued to divide his attention between giving dictation and viewing. Minutes passed until I could hold my tongue no longer. I interrupted and pointed out that unless we started our session immediately there would be no point in starting at all.

Two of the secretaries were instantly dismissed, leaving the one who had opened the door to me; she also happened to be the woman who had arranged the session. She was young and exceedingly attractive. Like her boss, she also wanted to quit smoking. I pulled up a chair. She sat directly opposite me, revealing even more length of leg than had already been generously displayed. At any other time I would have appreciated the view. On this occasion I could have done without the distraction.

Kerry remained stretched out watching Wimbledon. I commented that the television was a distraction.

'Geez! Can't I watch the tennis?'

The secretary switched off the set and told him to shut up and sit up. Without a murmur he did as he was told and the session began.

I always start by asking clients if we can use first names. Of the 25,000 people I have counselled personally, only one has ever objected, a dear old lady who asked me in the nicest way if I minded using her married name. From plain Joes and Janes to lords and ladies, none of the others have demurred. I had not the slightest hesitation in putting the same question to the national of a country that prides itself on its friendliness and informality. It's us Poms who are supposed to be the stuffed shirts, after all.

To my amazement he mulled over my request as though it was some complicated business deal. For both our sakes I avoided using his name altogether. I wish I had read Robert Maxwell's biography before I met Mr Packer. It would have given me valuable insight into the little tricks that some powerful men use to boost their self-esteem and keep everyone else firmly in their place.

I quickly realized that he was not taking in a word of the session, for every now and again I would hear him say: 'I don't want to be crook!' It wasn't so much an interruption as a sort of mantra repeated at intervals. I pointed out that he wasn't paying me to tell him what he already knew – that smoking was ruining his health. Obviously that was his main reason for wanting to quit, as it is for most smokers, but fear of being 'crook' was not going to make him quit. If that were the case he would have done it by now.

To his credit, once he accepted this point and the fact that he would have to start absorbing what I was telling him, he started listening rather than trying to dominate proceedings. Half an hour before the end of the allotted two hours, he suddenly stood up and interrupted my flow:

'You've done your job. I'm a non-smoker!'

This was a very good reaction and at that moment he truly was a non-smoker, but I had to ensure that the same positive frame of mind would last beyond our session and indeed remain for the rest of his life.

I said: 'I've not done yet.'

'Yes you have!'

He then turned to his secretary:

'Well, we can't smoke, so what shall we do?'

I was about to explain why it was important not to use substitutes – too late:

' I know, we'll celebrate with a bottle of Bollinger!'

It would have been futile to continue. Nothing I could say would get through to him. I gathered together my notes and belongings. As I did so, there was a loud thud as a fat bundle of bank notes landed in my briefcase.

I made my way back to Raynes Park accompanied by a jumble of angry thoughts. By the time I got home I felt completely drained, all thought of the fee gone until Joyce enquired as I ran through the evening's events. Together we counted the bundle of notes: £5,000. I could not get excited. I was too exhausted, anyway Packer was bound to ask for its return. No way could I see him succeeding as a result of my flying visit.

A few days later we received another call from his secretary:

'Kerry's started smoking again.'

It was the only time when news of a failure did not hurt me personally.

'He wants you to come back.'

I was prepared to try again but only on terms that would increase his chance of success and enable me to keep my temper.

I said: 'I'll gladly see him again, but I'm not going to waste his time or mine by coming out to him. He'll have to fix an appointment at my clinic.'

Needless to say, he didn't. Nor did he ask for the return of the £5,000. I subsequently discovered that his motto is, 'Never complain, never explain.'

Easyway's expansion has been due largely to personal recommendation. However, in recent years we have noticed an increase in the number of people coming to us as a result of stop-smoking campaigns initiated at work. In the early days it came as a pleasant surprise when I would get a string of people from the same organization. Obviously I was doing something right. But whether people came from a firm of brokers, such as Merrill Lynch, or from Wandsworth Prison, their experiences of smoking were remarkably similar.

Everyone comes to Easyway for the same reason, even people who might be regarded as being on the other side of the fence. When the marketing director of a large and famous tobacco company came to the clinic, my immediate reaction was to suspect his motives. Why on earth would he want a session? It turned out that he was the only member of his company's board who still smoked, and his fellow directors had put pressure on him to stop. Other employees from the same firm started booking sessions too. It soon became obvious that, like any other group of smokers, these people wanted to be free. I suppose it is logical. If you are a smoker, sooner or later you will want to escape from the trap, even if you make your living selling and promoting cigarettes.

The increase in the numbers of non-smokers is encouraging bosses to address the problems that arise with smokers in a work force. It is estimated that a smoker spends approximately 115 hours per year on unauthorized cigarette breaks, and takes at least 5 days more sick leave per year than non-smokers. In addition, smokers have 34 percent increased rate of absenteeism, 29 percent increased

risk of industrial injury, 40 percent increased risk of occupa-
tional injury, and 55 precent increased risk of disciplinary
action. The overall extra cost to a company of employing
just one smoker is estimated at more than £2000 per year. In
addition to the financial incentive for companies to
encourage smokers to quit, there is also the consideration of
improving relationships within their organization and
ending the segregation that often exists between smokers
and non-smokers. Not surprisingly, non-smokers resent the
extra breaks taken by their smoking colleagues, and the
higher rates of sickness and absenteeism.

Many companies approach us to help cure their workforce
of smoking either as part of an ongoing health initiative or
as a one off. Sessions are run for them at our clinics, on their
premises or at an off-site location of their choosing. One of
the first leading businessmen to make Easyway available to
his staff was Sir Richard Branson, who became convinced of
the effectiveness of the method and has since been a great
advocate of ours.

In the last few years Easyway has built an impressive
portfolio of corporate clients, including: Allied Dunbar,
Bayer AG, BMW, BP, British Airways, Citibank, Credit Suisse,
DHL, Du Pont, Ford, Guinness, Hewlett-Packard, Hilton
Hotels, IBM, IKEA, Inland Revenue, JP Morgan, Levi Strauss,
London Stock Exchange, Marks & Spencer, Microsoft,
Mobil, Nestlé, O2, Pfizer, PPP Healthcare, Proctor &
Gamble, Schweppes, Sony, Unilever and Woolworths.

This list continues to grow. It is interesting to note that, so
far, the corporate world has taken a positive view of
Easyway. It has done so because the method has worked for
enough of its employees to make it worthwhile continuing
to invest in sessions. There are two other powerful
institutions that might do well to follow their example.

Messaging the Media

It is said that there is no such thing as bad publicity. I would have to agree as I have been fortunate to receive wide coverage from the press and broadcast media. When I stepped aside to let Robin handle the expansion my intention was to spend my time spreading the word about Easyway. I was certain that the media would be a key ally in this.

I am always exceedingly nervous before an interview, not because I fear appearing foolish or even of being tongue-tied, but because I have a golden opportunity to spread an important message, and I desperately want to use the media time available to me to maximum advantage. This anxiety manifests itself as a frog in the throat. The first time it happened, I was in such a panic trying to shift it that I almost rendered myself speechless with choking. The problem persisted right up until the time we went on air, and then miraculously disappeared. The cause was obviously pure nerves, and I did not worry when it accompanied me on subsequent occasions. I knew it would go as soon as I was on air.

On the occasion of my interview with Selina Scott I arrived at the studio with my nerves jangling more than usual. I idolized her in exactly the same way as a youngster does a pop or film star. Deeply in love with her image, I was excited by the prospect of meeting her. It was routine to be met beforehand by a very attractive young woman who would offer refreshments and generally make me feel comfortable before I was whipped into position for the interview. The particular young woman who greeted me was blonde, exceptionally attractive and very attentive. She introduced me to the producer, the floor manager and various other people connected with the programme. I went through all of these niceties in a daze. All I could think of was whether I would be meeting Selina before the interview. I asked the question. There followed the longest pregnant pause of my life. Apart from the young woman, everyone in the room was staring at me with a look of abject disbelief, including Joyce. The young woman said:

'I am Selina Scott.'

I had imagined Selina to be on the tall side and I was expecting her to have shoulder-length hair. The young woman before me was quite short, as was her hair.

I understand there is a method of restraining a victim so that the more he tries to free himself the tighter the restraint becomes. With Selina Scott the more I tried to retrieve the situation, the worse it became. I have spent much of my life making *faux pas* and have learnt how to cover them up. But this time I was left speechless with humiliation at my blunder.

Despite this unfortunate start the programme went very well. Selina clearly wanted to get the best out of the interview for the benefit of her audience, and this in itself was gratifying.

As anti-matter is to matter, so Sod's law is to serendipity. Both have regularly punctuated my life. Just as the interview with Selina Scott was the one I most looked forward to and turned out to be the most embarrassing, so the one I was most dreading was in actuality one of the most agreeable. This interview was with LBC's Brian Hayes. I knew all about his phone-in because I used to listen to it regularly. I had him down as an exponent of a technique I call being humble to the mighty and mighty to the humble. Listening to his programme was like eavesdropping on people indulging in masochism. Regularly he would berate callers and then cut them off before they had a chance to defend themselves. Why I listened, I'm not quite sure. I can only assume it was in the hope that one day he would get his come-uppance. On several occasions he got me so irate that I rushed to the phone meaning to give him a piece of my mind, but I never managed to get through. When I received the invitation to be his special guest for a whole hour, Joyce counselled against acceptance:

'No way can you go. You know the effect he has on you.'

I was equally adamant. No way was I going to miss such a golden opportunity. Deep down, though, I felt very apprehensive. I arrived at the studio like the proverbial lamb awaiting slaughter.

My fears proved to be completely unfounded. Brian was charm and politeness personified, and very professional. He took the trouble to discuss the method with me before the programme and seemed to grasp the fundamentals quickly. When we came to the actual phone-in he did not, as I had feared he might, dominate the programme with his own ideas. He also has a wonderful facility for sussing out time-wasters quickly and despatching them even faster. True he doesn't suffer fools gladly, but then neither do I. I have had the pleasure of being interviewed by Brian several times, and on each occasion he has been highly constructive and a great asset to our cause.

One of the frustrating aspects of 'live' interviews is that rarely are you given warning of the questions you will be asked. LBC Radio's Bob Harris broke this rule. The interview was being given in the small hours. After a long day spent helping smokers to quit, I was feeling very tired. During the commercial break before my introduction, Bob said:

'I propose to start by asking you about the history of smoking and about the various chemicals that different tobacco companies include in their cigarettes.'

I explained that I had no more idea about the history of smoking than the next man, nor had I the slightest knowledge of the various chemicals that the tobacco companies include in their cigarettes. My only expertise was as the discoverer of a method that would enable any smoker to stop easily, immediately and permanently.

I was so relieved to have had the opportunity to set the record straight before we went on air. I sat there feeling confident that I would give a good account of myself. Bob went into his preamble:

'Tonight my guest is Allen Carr, who is an expert on smoking. Allen, can you start by giving us a brief history of smoking and telling us about the various chemicals that different tobacco companies include in their cigarettes.'

Once I recovered from the shock, I was tempted to fire back with: 'What sort of an idiot are you? I've just explained that I know nothing about the history of smoking and that my expertise is helping smokers to find it easy to quit. Why ask me a question I can't answer?'

How I wish I'd had the courage to say just that. I'm sure the listeners would have loved it. But I didn't. Instead I took a leaf out of the political canon of evasion and replied:

'I'm sure your listeners are no more interested in the history of smoking or the various chemicals that different tobacco companies put in their cigarettes than I am. However, I've a feeling they might be interested in the reason that LBC invited me here tonight – to explain just how easy it is to quit.'

The politician's ploy of dismissing a question as superficial and then proceeding to answer the question that suits his purpose proved to be very useful. Media time is precious, most of it – especially on television – being measured in seconds not minutes. I did not want to waste one of those precious seconds on issues that were not central to the subject of quitting smoking.

After an interview I am completely drained, annoyed with myself because I could have given more erudite answers or suspecting that I have dropped a clanger. I arrange to obtain recordings of the interviews but cannot bring myself to look at or listen to them for several days afterwards. When I do come to analyse them, they are never quite as bad as I had imagined. Giving interviews is rather like playing golf: you know you'll never achieve the perfect round, but you have to keep trying.

I would love a fiver for every interview or broadcast I have been asked to do on or around National No Smoking Day. As any smoker worth his salt will confirm, this is the one day in the year when he'll point blank refuse to quit. In fact smokers will smoke twice as much and twice as blatantly because they are sick and tired of being pilloried by society generally and particularly by those who have never smoked a cigarette in their lives.

However, it is also the one day in the year when Easyway can guarantee it will get a mention, just as the charities can be assured of publicity for the multitude of 'awareness' weeks that are jostling for media attention. Never mind that they spend the rest of the year in splendid isolation, completely forgotten except by the few whose lives are touched by or dedicated to them.

Invariably the first question put to me is, 'Why did you decide to give up?' It might just as well be, 'Why did you decide to duck when you realized the brick was about to hit your head?' This question is put in with the intention of prompting me to go into explicit detail about all the terrible effects of smoking, but it begs the question of who the programme makers are trying to help or inform.

Non-smokers are hardly likely to need reminding; they know smoking is self-destructive. The reaction of most smokers to having a litany of health risks recited to them is to reach for the 'Off' switch. I could never get programme makers to understand that the key issue with smoking is not the connection between smoking and lung cancer. This link has been established for over half a century, and is widely known, especially among smokers.

Indeed it seems that not a week goes by without some new health risk attaching to smoking. Almost without exception the programmes I have taken part in to discuss smoking have concentrated on this aspect, despite the demonstrable fact that it does not enable smokers to quit. Unfortunately, smoking is one of those issues that seems not to be deemed important enough to be treated seriously or to be given sufficient airtime to allow a proper discussion. The least satisfactory programmes in this respect are those with a star presenter feeding off the acclaim of a participating studio audience. Many of these programmes are just vehicles for self-display, for those on both sides of the footlights. Although cleverly done and presumably appealing to a wide audience, they do not succeed in even scratching the surface of the issues they purport to address, with 90 percent of the time spent on members of the audience either telling you it's impossible to quit or giving you a blow-by-blow account of how they did it. Everyone has a view, however inane. Often I will sit there thinking: 'Why have they invited me? Would a brain surgeon be expected to sit and listen to advice given by people who know nothing about the subject?' With brain surgery you have recognized experts and Joe Public. With quitting smoking everyone is an expert, even people who have never smoked.

One year TV-AM decided to launch a big anti-smoking campaign during the week leading up to National No Smoking Day, and asked me to take part. Paul Reisen was the man in charge of this campaign. I was delighted. It was the opportunity I had been waiting for. I had helped at least a dozen employees of TV-AM to quit successfully, and Paul Reisen happened to be one of them. He explained that each day they would be covering different methods of quitting and that he would like to feature my clinic on the final day. I said:

'Paul, you have personal proof that my system makes it easy to stop. Why don't you give me the whole week? I'll start a campaign that will get the whole world off smoking.'

He said: 'But some people can't do it the easy way. They have to do it the hard way.'

I started to explain that if people find it difficult to achieve their objective by doing it the easy way, they can not possibly improve their chances by making it harder.

He interrupted me:

'In any case, part of the campaign will be to go to the States to study their methods. They are always fifteen years ahead of us.'

. He was right. The United States usually is fifteen years ahead of us in most things, but in this one area they certainly are not. Easyway is light years ahead of any of their methods. Why else would smokers fly from all over the world, including the United States, for our sessions? I can understand Paul believing that the Americans might have something better to offer, but when he discovered they did not you might have hoped the producers would have insisted on revising the content of the programme.

One of the ground-breaking methods Paul brought to viewers involved smokers sitting in a tent together and singing, 'We're gonna give up smoking.' Asked how he was getting on, one of the participants, who had paid in the region of $1,000 for his 'treatment', replied: 'I haven't smoked a cigarette in four days and I can't wait to get out of here and light up!'

Easyway was featured on the final programme. Paul described how he had visited my clinic, paid £85, walked out four hours later already a non-smoker and had found it easy to stop. The plug did much to ease my frustration. However, any elation quickly disappeared when he finished the programme with:

'But you don't need to pay £85. If you really want to stop, you can do it yourself.'

Is any smoker likely to succeed if he doesn't want to quit? Of course not. The statement was made in the mistaken belief that, provided you want to quit, you will succeed. If people are capable of doing it themselves, why don't they? Why had the presenter himself sought my help? I could have understood his comment if he had quit after following his own advice. But, no, he had spent £85 and attended my clinic.

The vast majority of smokers have to find a key to unlock the door of the prison they are in. I spent over 30 years desperately wanting to quit but wanting was not sufficient to make me succeed. Easyway was the key that gave me my freedom, as it has millions of others.

Many smokers did contact me as a result of that programme, but I wonder how many others took its presenter's advice at face value and are still in the trap as a consequence.

The fact-sheet issued by TV-AM to accompany the campaign was par for the course and included information about a gimmick to help smokers quit: the 'Wrist-Flicker'. This consisted of a small piece of circular cardboard attached to an elastic band worn around the wrist. The idea was that every time the temptation to light up came upon the wearer, he or she would stretch the cardboard then let go and thus inflict pain. It was a depressing reminder of how far programme makers are prepared to sink and how far nicotine addiction has to go before it is accepted as the scourge it undoubtedly is. Would anyone dream of suggesting that a similar device be worn by heroin addicts?

You will think me either a glutton for punishment or one of the world's great optimists when I tell you that for NNSD 1992 I agreed to appear in another show devised by Paul Reisen. Called *The Last Cigarette*, it was a 90-minute extravaganza on how to quit. Given my previous experience, I should not have been so excited, but the bait was too alluring: over five minutes on national TV. I should have known better. Most of the programme was taken up with parading musicians, comedians and other celebrities.

As requested, I dutifully arrived at 8pm only to discover that I would not be required until nearly midnight. It would be a miracle if viewers had the stamina or patience to wait that long. As it turned out there was plenty going on in the waiting area to keep me amused. I came across John Stapleton, presenter of the consumer affairs programme, *Watchdog*, who was also scheduled to appear on the show. We got into conversation and he told me that he had attended our Raynes Park clinic nine months earlier and had not smoked since.

The trigger that inspired John to consult us was his wife's cancer. He had wanted to give her as much support as he could, and thought that the best way of doing this would be for him to stop smoking. He told me about an earlier failed attempt. This had been made as part of a television campaign when, apparently, umpteen million viewers had been charting his progress. Such circumstances might seem to provide a strong incentive for success, but clearly not strong enough.

I was interested to hear what John would tell the television audience, and thought the facts about his Easyway session were bound to figure. When his time came he explained that his success was due to his wife's cancer. End of story. I was baffled. The fact that he had succeeded when using Easyway but failed without it was highly relevant. He could have related the full story, including the fact that he had sought help, and let the audience make up its own mind as to the reason why he had succeeded. I have no doubt that his reason for wanting to stop was so he could support his wife, but if that motivation was actually responsible for his success, why had he needed to seek my help? I attributed it to a phenomenon of which we at Easyway are all too aware.

When they come to our clinics smokers are asked if they have tried other methods of quitting. Many say 'No'. During the therapy it transpires that many, including the 'Nos', have previously consulted not just one but several so-called experts. We also know that many ex-smokers who quit successfully after attending our clinics do not wish it to be known that they sought help and for this reason do not recommend us. Society believes that it takes willpower to stop smoking, and so regards anyone who seeks help to quit as weak-willed. Nobody wants to be put in this category, which is best avoided by denying that any help was sought. For people in the public eye, this attitude is perhaps especially understandable. It is also very damaging, ensuring that one of the principal myths about smoking is perpetuated.

I appeared on that show for about one minute at midnight, a minute shared with two other so-called experts. There was a doctor who spent the precious seconds explaining how marvellous a drug nicotine is; and a very pleasant lady who gave out tips on how to cope with the craving that smokers experience when they stop, a craving which she insisted lasts forever.

Life is too short to allow pride to get in the way of opportunity. I have long believed the media has the potential to get the truth about Easyway out to the general public, and so I was not prepared to refuse any further offers of exposure that might come my way. Some time after *The Last Cigarette* sank without trace, I was invited to appear on a TV programme called *The Time The Place*, with John Stapleton as presenter. The theme of this particular programme was the role parents who smoke play in influencing their children to smoke.

I could have told the programme makers that whether a parent smokes or not has absolutely no bearing whatsoever on whether their child will smoke. My father was a chain-smoker and most of my siblings were heavy smokers. For many years I believed that the need to smoke must be hereditary. I completely discounted the influence of my mother, who was a non-smoker and the dominant parent.

When I started the clinics I would ask each client if their parents smoked. If they did, the smoker would say: 'I obviously smoked because my parents did.' If the parents didn't, the smoker would say: 'I only started smoking to rebel against my parents.'

The tenor of the programme was unbearably pious. Apart from the poor devils who seemed to have been selected to provide cannon fodder, I was surrounded by holier-than-thou ex-smokers who were intent on making the smokers feel as uncomfortable and guilty as possible. Once again the programme seemed to be a missed opportunity, with the emphasis on the wrong aspect of smoking and ignoring the real problems confronting smokers when they try to quit. The plight of the smokers themselves was completely overlooked.

I talked to several of the smoking parents before the programme, and tried to give them as much advice about stopping as I could in the short time available to us. They were not ignorant, uncaring people. On the contrary, like most smoking parents, they openly admitted to feeling guilty about the example they were setting their children.

One pregnant 21-year-old was particularly sensitive to the charge that, because she had not stopped smoking, she was risking the health of her unborn child. The poor girl was virtually a child herself. She did not choose to fall into the trap. She wasn't smoking to kill her baby. She was smoking because she didn't know how to stop.

During the commercial break one couple said to me: 'We've taken in what you said and we've made up our minds to stop.' They told John of their decision. John relayed this information to the audience:

'We have some excellent news! Terry and Steve, having heard what they heard on this programme, said: "That's it, we're going to give up." You heard it here first, folks. Millions of you heard it on this programme. They don't smoke any more. Note particularly the people of Broughton, Salford and north-west England.'

I had not expected John to declare that my conversation with the couple had been in any way instrumental in their decision to try to quit. Before the programme he had told me that he could not mention Easyway because I make a charge for helping smokers to get free. However, I was surprised that he felt it necessary to alert the whole of north-west England, given his own experience of failing to stop when millions of viewers were following his progress. The more you try to pressurize smokers to stop, the more difficult you make their task.

I have no doubt that the intentions of most journalists and others in positions of informing public opinion are honourable. Their motivation is to serve truth and the public interest. My experience of journalists or opinion-formers falling below this standard is thankfully limited. On the whole, Easyway and I have received very fair coverage, which I like to think is an accurate reflection of our good reputation and the great many people we have succeeded in helping. The only time I have been moved to sue was when Virgin Radio's Chris Evans told his listeners that I had been seen lighting up.

I don't suppose he had any idea of the distress his comment would cause to the millions of smokers around the world who had quit smoking because of Easyway. My phone did not stop ringing for days. If I was smoking again, people told me, what hope was there for them? Chris Evans made his allegation in July 1999. In March 2001 he paid us costs and damages in an out of court settlement. Before the settlement Virgin Radio broadcast an apology. I hope that all the people who heard the lie also heard the retraction.

No doubt Chris Evans thought his comment was highly amusing and would entertain his audience. People don't regard smoking as a disease, so why should anyone object to poking fun at a man described variously as an 'anti-smoking guru' or as 'leading a one-man crusade against smoking'. Such labels suggest that I am some sort of crank or obsessive. I see myself as an ordinary man who has discovered a cure for smoking. If governments and doctors would recognize smoking as a disease and Easyway as the cure for it, millions of lives and a fortune in healthcare costs would be saved. I wonder what's stopping them?

Challenging the Establishment

I used to believe that when the benefits of Easyway became apparent, people in positions of authority – in government and in the health services – would advocate its use. After spending years trying to bring my method to their attention, I have reached the conclusion that their decisions in this regard must be based on factors unrelated to a qualitative assessment of the various quitting methods currently available. Why do I believe this?

Let me tell you about my experiences of the establishment bodies who are concerned with smoking as a public health issue, starting with the medical profession.

My first encounter with the mind-set of a representative bunch of doctors was at Worthing in the early Nineties when I was among several speakers invited by the local health authority to address the GPs in their area about methods of quitting. There was a doctor proclaiming the merits of acupuncture, a hypnotherapist, an expert in behavioural therapy, the inevitable representative of nicotine replacement therapy (NRT), and me.

In the course of their presentations the two other speakers emphasized the difficulties of quitting, confirmed that it required immense willpower, but that it was possible provided you had sufficient resolve to survive the prolonged misery. From memory, none of the other speakers claimed a success rate for their method in excess of 15 percent.

I was the last to speak. I had reason to be confident that the GPs would be impressed with Easyway. The officer of the health authority who had invited me to speak had already confirmed to the gathering that it had been recommended to her by several acquaintances and that, like them, she had quit with its help. The NRT representative had also been honest enough to inform everybody that his wife had quit successfully using Easyway. I outlined the advantages of the method over all others: no need for willpower, substitutes or any other gimmicks, no physical withdrawal pains, weight gain or a transitional period of misery, no feeling that social occasions would never be as enjoyable or that stressful situations would be impossible to handle. What's more the therapy was inexpensive, came with a money-back guarantee, and on the basis of that guarantee had a success rate in excess of 90 percent.

At the end, I invited questions. One man stood up. I looked at him expectantly, waiting for him to query some of my assertions. He declared that he couldn't see how my method was any better than the others.

Baffled by the general lack of interest, and not a little aggrieved by his remark, I let my irritation show:

'I assume you have been listening to the same speakers as I have. They have confirmed how difficult it is to quit, how much willpower is needed, how long it takes, how miserable smokers feel. They've also admitted the chances of a smoker succeeding using their methods are not great: they quoted a success rate of less than 15 percent. I've been describing a method that is immediate, permanent and easy, which requires no willpower whatsoever and has a success rate of over 90 percent. I can understand why you might question my claims, but I cannot comprehend how you fail to see the difference between my method and theirs.'

The GP did not bother to respond, and as no one else wanted to take the discussion forward, we broke for refreshments. During this interlude another doctor came up to me and commented that I must have formed the impression that he and his fellow GPs were wearing blinkers. I couldn't disagree with him. He went on to explain that helping smokers to quit is just one of the many problems a GP has to cope with, that there was not the time to investigate other methods and it was so much easier to prescribe NRT. In any case, smoking is a self-inflicted disease and if smokers choose to ignore medical advice to quit, they have only themselves to blame.

My youngest son, Richard, is a doctor. I know something of the burdens imposed by patient expectations, long hours and too much paperwork. It is hardly surprising that many GPs prefer to spend the little time available to them helping people who are not bent on destroying their health. Nor is ignorance of the subject of smoking uncommon. Most doctors don't know about the advantages or disadvantages of the various quitting methods. The irony is that doctors are held up to be the experts. People expect them to know. In all my TV appearances where there was a doctor among the guests, viewers would be referred to him at the end of the programme if they needed any 'help' or 'information'. Invariably the doctor would advocate nicotine gum, and invariably he would be antagonistic towards me because I was advocating Easyway.

I remember after one broadcast, a doctor turning to me

and saying accusingly: 'You charge a fee to help smokers stop.'

I charge a fee just as anybody else who provides a service charges a fee. I make no apologies for that. If we lived in a society that used pebbles as currency, I would receive pebbles, as would everybody else. Some time later I learned that the same doctor was being paid to plug nicotine substitutes.

The reality is that doctors are working within a very narrow band of knowledge handed down to them from public health officials higher up the chain who have decided to adopt a particular policy on smoking. In some instances doctors are simply peddling products supplied directly to them by the pharmaceuticals industry. In Britain the National Health Service spends about £1,000 to get a smoker to stop for one month. We have offered all NHS Primary Care Trusts our services at a tenth of that cost, with the additional benefit of our money-back guarantee. Our offer has been turned down.

Since the introduction of publicly funded stop-smoking programmes, two questionable methods have been given the full backing of the medical establishment: willpower and NRT.

I have explained at length elsewhere why willpower doesn't work. NRT may sound very plausible, and seem to offer a means of escaping two of the most powerful mythical consequences of any attempt to quit smoking. The myth purveyors insist that, in order for an attempt to succeed, the smoker must defeat two formidable opponents: the habit itself and the terrible physical pains that accompany nicotine withdrawal. Few boxers could beat Mohammed Ali in his prime, and Rocky Marciano remained undefeated throughout his entire career as world heavyweight champion. Only a fool or a madman would have contemplated taking on two Alis or two Marcianos at the same time. Similar reasoning informs the use of NRT. The smoker first takes on the habit, by stopping smoking but keeping the body supplied with nicotine in the form of gum, a patch, spray or lozenge. Once the habit has been broken, he takes on the withdrawal pains, gradually reducing his nicotine intake.

Many doctors involved in the treatment of heroin addiction question the sense in giving addicts a substitute such as methadone, which is in itself addictive. I question the sense in giving NRT to nicotine addicts. True, users are not ingesting all those fumes and tar, but they are still absorbing the substance to which they have become addicted. It is ironic that governments and the medical profession, many of whom agree that nicotine addiction is at the root of the problem with smoking, insist on the banning of tobacco advertising and yet are content to promote the consumption of nicotine in another form.

NRT is one of the big ideas – and big money spinners – of the pharmaceuticals industry. When it was originally developed, in the 1970s by a subsidiary of Swedish Tobacco Company, it was intended as a tobacco substitute for sub-mariners who for obvious reasons were forbidden to smoke when their vessels were submerged. Only in the last twenty years has it been touted as an aid to quitting. Unfortunately, smokers believe they get pleasure from smoking and so it seems perfectly logical to them to try NRT. They don't make the connection between their dependency and nicotine. They also believe they won't be able to cope with the terrible withdrawal symptoms associated with quitting, and indeed this is the main 'use' of NRT, according to its makers. They might just as well be honest and tell smokers that the purpose of NRT is to keep them hooked on nicotine. I am amazed that no one has questioned the accuracy of the term Nicotine Replacement Therapy. What is being replaced? Certainly not nicotine, as even a cursory scrutiny of the ingredients of these products reveals.

In our clinics we see people who have used NRT to try to wean themselves off cigarettes. All they have succeeded in doing is changing their system of delivering nicotine. Instead of a cigarette they now use patches, lozenges or gum to keep their body topped up. In some cases, people have gone back to smoking cigarettes as well as taking NRT, so they are getting nicotine from two separate sources.

The latest quit-smoking product is Zyban, containing the drug bupropion, which was first developed to treat depression. By altering the levels of some chemicals in the brain, it is said to relieve those mythical withdrawal symptoms. Zyban is a prescription medicine and comes with a list of precautions. Side effects associated with it can include nausea, vomiting, abdominal pain, insomnia, tremor, concentration disturbance, headache, dizziness, anxiety, rash, sweating and taste disorders.

The relationship between the pharmaceutical conglomerates and the medical profession has grown increasingly incestuous over the years as our drug culture has developed. By drug culture I mean our reliance on synthetic medicines. I have great admiration for many of the cures now possible with modern drug technology. However to use such technology in the battle to stop people smoking is a waste of scarce resources. In spring 2003 the manufacturers of Zyban took legal action when the Australian Pharmaceutical Advisory Benefits

Committee tried to impose new controls on the treatment because of concerns over its cost and effectiveness. One group of researchers reported that, although bupropion had been prescribed to 10 percent of Australian smokers, this had had no obvious effect on the prevalence of smoking.

Smoking is widely perceived as a medical problem. It's not. If it were, Easyway would not be a successful cure for it. The diseases related to smoking are medical problems, but the activity itself and why people do it are not.

Smoking cessation is seen by the pharmaceuticals industry as a growth area for their business, and so they are prepared to invest, not just in research and development but also in well targeted promotion, such as sponsoring the 10th World Conference on Tobacco or Health. That said, I did get an invitation to it, by way of one of those serendipitous happenings that have occurred throughout my life. Ted Thomas, a journalist, businessman and long-term resident of Hong Kong, contacted me after he heard an interview I gave on LBC.

He was struck by the indisputable logic of Easyway and, having recently lost a number of close friends to smoking-related diseases, was moved to ask me if I would set up a clinic in his adopted homeland.

I was more than happy to accept the challenge. I could not pass up an opportunity to spread the Easyway message, and I had long wanted to see Hong Kong. What a glorious coincidence of pleasures – and so it proved.

Joyce and I were installed in a luxury hotel overlooking the bay and treated like royalty. This was a few years before Britain's lease expired and the island was handed back to China. We experienced a kind of lifestyle that must have been close to what was routine in the days of the British Raj. We were thoroughly pampered, and enjoyed every minute of it, especially Joyce who managed to purchase at least 50 percent of the contents of Stanley Market during our stay. Even the 'work' aspect was exceedingly pleasant. The clinic was held in an outbuilding of the Matilda hospital, perched atop Hong Kong's famous peak. The views were spectacular and I could think of no location more suited to assisting smokers to quit and convincing them that there is a great life to be had without tobacco.

One of the main pluses to come out of our visit was my meeting with Dr Judith Mackay, Director of the Asian Consultancy on Tobacco Control and the leading anti-smoking campaigner in South East Asia. Like me, she takes pride in being a thorn in the side of Big Tobacco; she regards it as a particular honour to have been identified by the tobacco industry as one of the three most dangerous people in the world. I was flattered that Judith was interested in meeting me. In truth, she wanted to become better acquainted with my method and asked if she might sit in on a session. Several of her acquaintances had quit because of Easyway, all of them heavy smokers whom Judith had given up as lost causes.

For anyone who genuinely wants to quit smoking, an Easyway session can be both an enlightening and exhila-rating experience. For an observer, especially a non-smoker, it must be as interesting as reading the instructions for assembling a model aircraft kit, without having the slightest intention of actually putting the contraption together. After sitting through four four-hour sessions, Judith had to admit that she could not fathom how the method works. Not knowing the answer to this question has never bothered me nor, presumably, the thousands of other people it has saved from nicotine addiction. I would discover, however, that it matters a great deal to the public health officials who decide upon which quit-smoking methods to support.

As one of the conference organizers of the 10th World Conference on Tobacco or Health, Judith was instrumental in arranging my invitation. The year was 1997, in the month following the historic handing back of Hong Kong to China, the place Beijing. I considered the invitation one of the biggest honours in my life. These conferences had previously been the sole preserve of academics, scientists and government officials, and for me it was a golden opportunity to get Easyway recognized by the international health community. In addition to almost 900 'experts' on smoking and tobacco control from 101 countries, there was a contingent of some 800 Chinese working in the same areas.

My invitation included the opportunity to give a talk on Easyway. Unlike at home, I would not be dealing with GPs whose knowledge of smoking was limited, but experts specializing in the subject. During the five days of the conference Robin and I sat through lecture after lecture. Many of the speakers came across as being there principally to justify their position at the top table of the anti-smoking establishment. Without exception, these speakers highlighted two main areas of concern. The first was the carnage that smoking is causing throughout the world: 3.5 million tobacco-related deaths in 1997, increasing to 10 million by 2025, with 7 million of these deaths occurring in developing countries and 50 percent of them occurring between the ages of 35 and 69. I suppose with statistics like these it would not have been sensible to proclaim that the programmes in place were working well. After detailing the litany of problems existing in his particular area, each speaker concluded by saying that more research was needed. Research for what? To break down the statistics over different, cultures, religions or professions? What would that prove? We already know that smoking is the world's No 1 killer disease. All we really need is a cure.

I was still naive enough to believe that these dedicated medical experts would want to hear about Easyway. Unfortunately, my talk turned out to be a dialogue of the deaf. I suppose I am not used to 'presenting' my method in a form that scientists understand. I spend too much time dealing with real people in the real world. I could not provide the sort of details and data required by my august audience. It was an intensely frustrating experience and I have to admit to losing my cool on several occasions. Fortunately Judith did not hold this mutual failure in communication and understanding against me. I am immensely grateful for her continuing support for Easyway. She is a true ally. It is a great pity there are not many more Judith Mackays in the public health establishment, people who are committed to doing the right thing and are not intent on pushing their own agenda.

In the public health arena it is unfortunately true that value for money – in terms of what actually works – tends to play second fiddle to what has become established practice. It is understandably difficult for people who have spent perhaps 20 years of their lives tackling a problem in one way to accept that they have been going about it in the wrong way. When someone like me comes along and points this out, it is easier to ignore or deride the messenger than institute change. At times I have become depressed by this attitude and seriously wondered whether my goal of making Easyway available to every smoker is not doomed to failure.

I have been encouraged recently by the news that BUPA and PPP Healthcare, the two largest private healthcare companies in the UK, are to offer Easyway to their corporate clients. We have had similar endorsement in Germany, too, with the German Association of Corporate Health Insurers (BKK), the country's third largest, giving its roughly ten million members the right to claim a contribution for an Easyway session. In the past therapists without a recognized medical qualification have been ignored by health insurers. Easyway is regarded as a special case, which is testimony to the method's effectiveness.

At the end of *The Easy Way to Stop Smoking*, I wrote:

'There is a wind of change in society. A snowball has started that I hope this book will turn into an avalanche.'

15th July 2003 was the 20th anniversary of my discovery of Easyway. As I write, in global terms I estimate that I have helped to expand that snowball to the size of a football. Not exactly outstanding success after 20 years, you might think, particularly as I have had the assistance of so many intelligent, industrious and dedicated people. Nevertheless I am proud of our achievements and combined efforts to date.

Although I might not personally live to see that avalanche, eventually advocates of Easyway will. How can I be so positive? Because the truth will out, and once it is out it will not be shushed into silence. Only in the last 500 years of the existence of human life on this planet has it generally been accepted that the Earth is round not flat. Experts have throughout history got major facts wrong.

Unfortunately, as with some giant super-tanker, once a course is set it takes time to turn opinion round, especially when vested interests and reputations are at stake. Wrong thinking becomes embedded in minds closed to change or even reappraisal.

In the not too distant future, smoking will be thought of as one of those things we used to do. And I am convinced Easyway will have played a large part in bringing this about. Events will overtake the decision makers. As often happens in life, people will find the means of their own salvation where smoking is concerned – and choose Easyway to help them.

Epilogue

Watching someone make the transition from smoker to non-smoker is, for me, about as satisfying as life gets. There is a saying about being a victim of one's own success. In one sense that happened to me with the expansion of Easyway, which meant it was no longer feasible for me to spend 99 percent of my time working with clients. Instead I became involved in writing books, giving interviews and, the most satisfying aspect of my new role, corresponding with problem smokers.

I don't like writing books, being interviewed, travelling or staying in hotels. And I positively loathe being photographed. All in all, I am the world's most reluctant front man. But, I make no complaint about fulfilling those unloved functions. They are part of a debt of gratitude I can never repay.

Because of Easyway, I was released from two self-imposed incarcerations: accountancy and slavery to nicotine. Without it I would not have enjoyed the happiness and excitement of the last 20 years or be able to look forward to enjoying so much more. I would have looked back on my life as a precious gift wasted.

However, without the experience of being both an unhappy accountant and a smoker, I could never have unravelled the mysteries of nicotine addiction. In life adversity and bad experiences have the potential to convert waste into preparation for achievement, so long as we learn the lessons they offer us.

All addictions do us a disservice, and not just in health terms. Because of them we hide from ourselves and avoid confronting the illusions that bind us to destructive types of behaviour and limiting ways of seeing the world. One of the tenets of Easyway is, 'Don't use substitutes'. Smoking can become a substitute for life itself. While we remain hooked, we fail to appreciate the many causes for celebration around us.

I think of myself as luckier than any man has a right to be. Luck, good fortune, call it what you will, is available to everyone. My name for it is serendipity. I am a true believer in this phenomenon, which I only began to take seriously after that revelatory turning point 20 years ago. With Joyce it has been my constant companion ever since. Work with it and you too will find it is a generous provider.

Index